ADVANCES IN VIRAL ONCOLOGY

Volume 6

Advances in Viral Oncology
Volume 6

*Experimental Approaches to Multifactorial
Interactions in Tumor Development*

Editor

George Klein, M.D., D.Sc.

*Department of Tumor Biology
Karolinska Institutet
Stockholm, Sweden*

Raven Press ❦ New York

Raven Press, 1185 Avenue of the Americas, New York, New York 10036

Made in the United States of America
987654321

Library of Congress Cataloging-in-Publication Data
Main entry under title:

Experimental approaches to multifactorial
   interactions in tumor development.

   (Advances in viral oncology; v. 6)
   Includes bibliographies and index.
   1. Carcinogenesis.   2. Viral carcinogenesis.
3. Oncogenes.   4. Cancer—Genetic aspects.
I. Klein, George, 1925–   II. Series.
[DNLM: 1. Cell Transformation. Neoplastic.
2. Oncogenes.   W1 AD888 v.6 / QZ 202 E958]
RC268.5.E98   1986   616.99′4071   86-26038
ISBN 0-88167-190-8

Preface

Peyton Rous first defined tumor progression as the process by which tumors "go from bad to worse."[1] Leslie Foulds widened the concept and defined its rules, based on a judicious combination of descriptive and experimental analysis of the natural history of cancer in man and in animals.[2] The multistep nature of cancer development was also suggested by the statistical analysis of the age-incidence curves for most of the major human cancers that arise in adults.[3]

Foulds' analysis has led to the important concept of "unit characteristics" i.e., cancer-related phenotypic traits that together compose the very real but nevertheless elusively ill-definable entity known as the malignant cell, without being exclusively or even regularly associated with every one of its protean manifestations. Foulds' "units" relate to growth rate, hormone dependence, invasiveness, and also to some more complex behavioral traits, such as the ability to metastasize or to grow in free-floating ascites rather than the firmly anchored, solid form.[3,4] Our current language uses somewhat different terms, such as "immortalization," changes in contact relationships or other aspects of intercellular behavior *in vitro,* serum requirements, or, increasingly, dependence on a growth factor, and specific differentiation blocks—*plus ça change, plus c'est la même chose.* The neoplastic evolution is still most adequately described in Foulds' terminology as the result of multiple stepwise changes in one or several unit characteristics that reassort themselves independently of each other and thereby create the impression of a process that moves along alternative pathways, leading to individually distinct phenotypic patterns in different tumors. The underlying process of clonal and subclonal variation and selection[4] must act by favoring the gradual emancipation of the cell, step by step, from the growth limitations in the original host environment. Tumorigenicity is the most visible manifestation of this process, but it is not the final stage. Autonomy is never total, and progression has no endpoint, as Foulds repeatedly pointed out. Even the most highly malignant tumors can extend the range of their ability for progressive growth (e.g., to include new tissue compartments, more unfavorable hormonal environments, or new host genotypes.)

Because division of somatic cells is regulated by the internal program of the cell and by multiple host controls operated by both positive and negative regulatory signals, the emancipation of the neoplastic clone must necessarily proceed through several steps.

[1]P. Rous and J. W. Beard, *J. Exp. Med,* 62:523–548 (1935).
[2]L. Foulds, *J. Chron. Dis.,* 8:2–37 (1958).
[3]For review, see E. Farber and R. Cameron, *Adv. Cancer Res.,* 31:125–226 (1980).
[4]G. Klein and E. Klein, *Symp. Soc. Exp. Biol.,* 11:305–328 (1957).

Is there, then, nothing new under the sun? Yes and no. The natural history of cancer and its phenotypic description have remained the same, but there is important news that concerns the genetic level. The unexpected gift of viral oncology to cellular biology, the discovery of the oncogenes, and the subsequent development of molecular biology have put us in a position where it is possible to define, isolate, clone, and sequence some of the genes that can transform normal cells to neoplastic cells, provided that the cells are "ready to jump" (i.e., when their own program, the expression of other genes, and the actual environment so permits).

The first volume of this series (*Oncogene Studies*, published in 1982) dealt with the basic information on most of the major oncogene groups. The list of known oncogenes has not increased to any major extent since then. This is in line with the frequently expressed view that the number of potential oncogenes is probably limited. There has been much progress in defining their biological activity in the cell, including both normal and pathological manifestations at the phenotypic level. Their complementary interactions in transformation and tumorigenicity are particularly relevant for this volume. One of the major surprises has been to watch how smoothly the extrinsic, parasitic, and seemingly quite alien DNA tumor viruses have melted into the landscape of the intrinsic, cell-derived oncogenes that have been brought to us by the RNA tumor viruses with their totally different life style. The repeated demonstration that the highly artificial transfection experiment with tumor-derived DNA can lead to *in vitro* transformation and even tumorigenicity in susceptible target cells across tissue and species barriers and that this activity is partly due to some of the same oncogenes (*ras* in particular) that had been identified by the classical viral transduction models was another surprise. The third, and perhaps most unexpected, window has been opened by an experiment of nature, recognized as the illegitimate activation of some of the same oncogenes (*myc* in particular) by chromosomal translocations. This cytogenetically recognizable event is regularly involved in the genesis of certain tumors that arise from a given cell type (most frequently B-lymphocytes), and it can show surprisingly precise homologies between different species. The amplification of some oncogenes (particularly *myc*) that may occur in the course of tumor progression, usually as a late event, is the fourth surprise that has been encountered in this veritable wonderland during the past few years.

Is there no exception from the rule of multistep evolution in cancer? The one major exception comes from the virally transduced oncogenes. Some of them, v-*src* in particular, can transform normal into malignant cells *in vitro* and *in vivo* in a single step. However, as Temin[5] has repeatedly pointed out, the v-*onc* sequences have evolved through many serial passages, performed by investigators under continuous selection for high transforming ability and/or tumorigenicity. This is very different from spontaneous tumor development, where selection acts on the cell and favors single changes in multiple genes. The products of the v-*onc* genes act as multifunctional proteins that can influence the cell at several different

---

[5]H. Temin, *J. Cell Physiol.*, 3:1–11 (1984).

levels, in analogy with the complementary effects of different oncogenes in the usual *in vitro* models. The viral pickup of two unrelated and unlinked oncogenes that act in a complementary fashion, reviewed by Klaus Bister in this volume, illustrates the power of this selection in its most clearly visible form. It is less easy to understand how exogenous DNA viruses, with polyoma as the best explored example, could have acquired the capacity to code for similarly interacting proteins and even conserve some of them in a double code, disentangled by alternative splicing and frameshift. Is this a side effect of the viral strategy, a consequence of the evolution that has led to moderate interactions between the virus and the host cell and prolonged latency? The unexpected discovery that exogenous, DNA-viral "transforming genes" can replace certain oncogenes and complement the transforming function of others may open the way toward an understanding of the common features of latency and transformation.

Is the activation of oncogenes by viruses, mutations, translocations, or gene amplification the major and perhaps the only key to the understanding of tumor development and progression? Certainly not. Although they are in the focus of most current attention, the oncogenes represent only one of at least three major worlds of genes that can influence neoplastic behavior. The second world comprises the tumor suppressor genes or "antioncogenes." The third world may be referred to as modifier genes. They are not directly involved in tumorigenesis (or its prevention) but may modulate metastatic behavior (like the major histocompatibility complex) or invasiveness (e.g., by controlling cell adhesion or proteolytic activity).

The tumor-suppressor genes are beginning to take shape, as also reflected by several articles in this volume. Their inactivation or loss may turn out to be as important for the multistep development of tumors as the activation of the oncogenes. The somatic hybridization experiments, reviewed by Eric J. Stanbridge, demonstrate that some suppressor genes may act by providing the neoplastic cell with the capacity for terminal differentiation in an appropriate *in vivo* environment. The revertant analysis of Robert H. Bassin and Makoto Noda shows that cellular genes may impose a quasi-normal phenotype on the v-*ras*-transformed cell, in spite of the continued expression of the originally transforming oncogene protein at the same level. Somatic hybridization of such revertants with cells transformed by a variety of oncogenes has shown that some will be suppressed while others remain transformed, depending on the oncogene. This is probably the first oncogene-related functional study of a suppressor system. Similar studies may help to elucidate the transforming mechanisms of oncogenes from a new angle.

Blocking of specific differentiation steps has been a recurrent theme in tumor development. Studies on temperature-sensitive v-*onc* mutants have been particularly informative in showing that these oncogenes may act by imposing specific blocks to myoblast, chondrocyte, or melanoblast differentiation (for v-*src*) or erythroid differentiation (for v-*erb*-B).[6] It appears to be a general rule from these ex-

---

[6]For review, see G. Klein and E. Klein, Conditioned tumorigenicity of activated oncogenes. *Cancer Res.*, 46:3211-3224(1986).

periments that the characteristic differentiation products of each phenotype fail to be expressed at the permissive temperature but may appear promptly when the oncogene is temporarily switched off by a temperature shift. Return to the permissive temperature leads to full reexpression of the oncogene, but this can no longer prevent the progress of the cell along its original differentiation program. This is in line with the widely affirmed concept that activated oncogenes can only transform and/or contribute to the tumorigenic process if expressed in cells positioned at specific windows of differentiation.

The interplay between activated oncogenes that favor proliferation in certain cell types and the effect of external signals and internal programs that control differentiation must be finely poised in each cell. Imbalanced cell populations, biased toward growth rather than differentiation, can often be influenced by appropriate differentiation-inducing signals, as illustrated by the article of Leo Sachs on myeloid leukemia. Similar scenarios will no doubt follow for many other tumors that respond to differentiation induction, such as teratoma, erythroleukemia, and histiocytoma. This is an important area, since a detailed understanding of differentiation-inducing factors and cellular responsiveness may provide pivotal information for therapeutic interventions based on physiological mechanisms.

This volume reviews some of the experimental approaches to the problem of multifactorial interactions in tumor development. A subsequent volume (Volume 7) deals with the analysis of some actual multistep scenarios in the natural history of cancer.

This volume will be of interest to all research oncologists, as well as to virologists, immunologists, and cellular and molecular biologists.

GEORGE KLEIN

Acknowledgment

The Editor would like to express his gratitude to all authors for their painstaking work.

Contents

1   **Analysis of Malignant Phenotypes by Oncogene Complementation**
H. Earl Ruley

21   **Stepwise Transformation and Cooperative Interactions Involving Oncogenes of DNA Tumor Viruses**
F. Cuzin and G. Meneguzzi

45   **Multiple Cell-Derived Sequences in Single Retroviral Genomes**
Klaus Bister

71   **Sequences that Influence the Transforming Activity and Expression of the *mos* Oncogene**
George F. Vande Woude, Marianne Oskarsson, Mary Lou McGeady, Arun Seth, Friedrich Propst, Martin Schmidt, Richard Paules, and Donald G. Blair

83   **Genetic Regulation of Tumorigenic Expression in Somatic Cell Hybrids**
Eric J. Stanbridge

103   **Oncogene Inhibition by Cellular Genes**
Robert H. Bassin and Makoto Noda

129   **Development and Suppression of Malignancy**
Leo Sachs

143   **Oncogenes, Genetic Instability, and Evolution of the Metastatic Phenotype**
Garth L. Nicolson

169   **Subject Index**

Contributors

Robert H. Bassin

Laboratory of Tumor Immunology and
  Biology
National Cancer Institute
Bethesda, Maryland 20892

Klaus Bister

Otto-Warburg-Laboratorium
Max-Planck-Institut für Molekulare Genetik
D-1000 Berlin 33 (Dahlem)
Federal Republic of Germany

Donald G. Blair

LBI-Basic Research Program
NCI-Frederick Cancer Research Facility
P. O. Box B
Frederick, Maryland 21701

F. Cuzin

Laboratoire de Génétique Moléculaire des
  Papovavirus
Inserm U-273
Centre de Biochemie
Parc Valrose
06034 Nice, France

George Klein

Department of Tumor Biology
Karolinska Institute
Box 60400
104 01 Stockholm, Sweden

Mary Lou McGeady

LBI-Basic Research Program
NCI-Frederick Cancer Research Facility
P. O. Box B
Frederick, Maryland 21701

G. Meneguzzi

Laboratoire de Génétique Moléculaire des
  Papovavirus
Inserm U-273
Centre de Biochemie
Parc Valrose
06034 Nice, France

Garth L. Nicolson

Department of Tumor Biology
The University of Texas
M. D. Anderson Hospital and Tumor
  Institute
Houston, Texas 77030

Makoto Noda

The Institute of Physical and Chemical
  Research
Wako, Saitama 351-01, Japan

Marianne Oskarsson

LBI-Basic Research Program
NCI-Frederick Cancer Research Facility
P. O. Box B
Frederick, Maryland 21701

Richard Paules

LBI-Basic Research Program
NCI-Frederick Cancer Research Facility
P. O. Box B
Frederick, Maryland 21701

Freidrich Propst

LBI-Basic Research Program
NCI-Frederick Cancer Research Facility
P. O. Box B
Frederick, Maryland 21701

H. Earl Ruley

Center for Cancer Research and
  Department of Biology
Massachusetts Institute of Technology
Cambridge, Massachusetts 02139

Leo Sachs

Department of Genetics
Weizmann Institute of Science
Rehovot 76100, Israel

Martin Schmidt

LBI-Basic Research Program
NCI-Frederick Cancer Research Facility
P. O. Box B
Frederick, Maryland 21701

Arun Seth
LBI-Basic Research Program
NCI-Frederick Cancer Research Facility
P. O. Box B
Frederick, Maryland 21701

Eric J. Stanbridge
Department of Microbiology
& Molecular Genetics

College of Medicine
University of California, Irvine
Irvine, California 92717

George F. Vande Woude
LBI-Basic Research Program
NCI-Frederick Cancer Research Facility
P. O. Box B
Frederick, Maryland 21701

Advances in Viral Oncology, Volume 6, edited by
George Klein. Raven Press, New York © 1987.

Analysis of Malignant Phenotypes by Oncogene Complementation

H. Earl Ruley

Center for Cancer Research and Department of Biology,
Massachusetts Institute of Technology,
Cambridge, Massachusetts 02139

Oncogenes are genes implicated in carcinogenesis by virtue of their associations with oncogenic viruses and tumor-specific chromosome abnormalities and by their ability to transform cultured cells to a tumorigenic state (7,25,53). Oncogenes manifest biologically dominant phenotypes as a result of activating mutations and virus associations. These biological activities have allowed oncogenes to be molecularly cloned and analyzed with regard to gene structure and mechanisms of activation.

Understanding how oncogenes transform cells will require characterizing biochemical activities of oncogene proteins and metabolic pathways altered by these activities and determining how these pathways influence cell growth and differentiation. Although difficulties in manipulating mammalian cells preclude the types of genetic analysis possible with simpler organisms, genetic approaches offer the best means of unraveling interactions among biochemical activities responsible for oncogenic phenotypes. To this end, recent studies have used cloned oncogenes to identify situations where transformation by one oncogene requires activities supplied by a second oncogene. The observed collaborations suggest that certain oncogenes express complementing biochemical activities that enable other oncogenes to transform cultured cells.

This article reviews several experimental systems in which oncogenic transformation appears to require two or more complementing oncogenes. We shall consider the possible significance of oncogene interactions and how interactions of this type may be exploited to study oncogene functions.

ONCOGENE COMPLEMENTATIONS

That two or more oncogenes might express complementing activities required for cell transformation was first suggested by studies with polyoma virus and with human adenoviruses. In particular, activities of two or more viral polypeptides were required to transform cultured primary cells to a tumorigenic state. These could be supplied either by two adenovirus early transcription units, E1A and E1B [reviewed in Van der Eb and Bernards (52)] or by the small, middle, and large tumor antigens encoded by the polyoma virus early region (35). By contrast, activities of the polyoma virus middle T antigen were sufficient to transform cells from several established lines (35,50). Finally, both adenovirus E1A and the polyoma virus large T antigen expressed activities that enabled certain primary cells to escape senescence and grow indefinitely in culture as established cell lines (17,36). Together, these observations suggested that transformation of cultured primary cells could require at least two complementing activities that separately facilitate *in vitro* establishment and conversion to a tumorigenic phenotype.

These studies led two groups to investigate the question of oncogene complemention further (24,38). Several laboratories had isolated cellular oncogenes from human tumor cells related to the *ras* oncogenes, identified in association with murine retroviruses (7,25). The oncogenic potentials of cellular *ras* genes were greatly enhanced by point mutations resulting in single amino acid substitutions (53). Since activating mutations enabled *ras* oncogenes to transform cells from the established NIH3T3 line, it was particularly interesting to determine whether activated *ras* genes expressed activities sufficient to transform cultured primary cells.

Figure 1 illustrates results obtained in our laboratory using primay baby rat kidney (BRK) cells (38). As expected, neither the polyoma virus middle T antigen *(pmt)* nor adenovirus E1B individually induced transformed foci on BRK monolayers. Similarly, the *ras* oncogene cloned from T24 bladder carcinoma cells was also unable to transform primary BRK cells. By contrast, all three oncogenes induced transformed foci when cotransfected with adenovirus type 2 E1A. A normal Ha-*ras* 1 gene did not transform even when cotransfected with E1A, indicating that oncogene activation, although necessary, was not sufficient for transformation of primary BRK cells.

In similar experiments, *ras* oncogenes transformed secondary rat embryo fibroblast (REF) cells (24) or Syrian hamster embryo cells (47); however, the resulting transformants were not tumorigenic and usually senesced after a limited number of population doublings. By contrast, plasmids encoding the polyoma virus large T antigen *(plt),* the v-*myc* oncogene of MC29 virus, and a transcriptionally activated c-*myc* gene collaborated with the Ha-*ras* oncogene to convert embryonic fibroblasts to a tumorigenic phenotype.

E1A, *myc,* and *plt* individually did not transform cultured BRK or REF cells, but induced clones of cells that had extended growth potential compared with untransfected primary cells (17,30,36,40). These cells gave rise to established lines capable of growing indefinitely *in vitro* but lacked properties of oncogenically transformed cells, such as the ability to grow in soft agar or to form tumors in animal hosts. As shown in Fig. 2, enhanced growth of BRK cells transfected by the v-*myc* oncogene of MC29 virus was indicated by the ability to form colonies in dilute culture (40). Cells within these colonies were easily expanded to mass culture and grew continuously without crisis as established lines. By contrast, un-

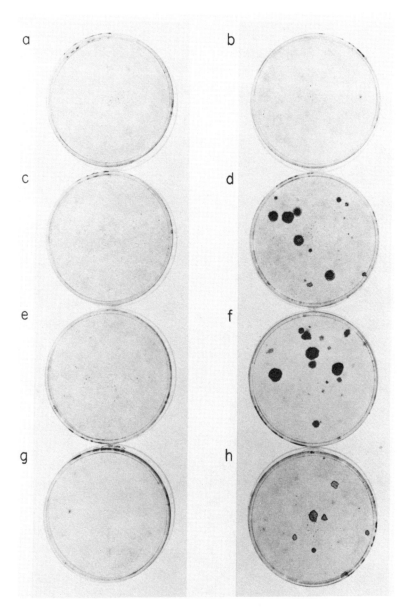

FIG. 1. Focus assay following transfection of baby rat kidney cells by transforming genes alone or with Ad-2 E1A. Cells were transfected with viral genes and cellular oncogenes and stained with Giemsa at various times thereafter: **(a)** no plasmid; **(b)** Ad-2 E1A; **(c)** T24 Ha-*ras* 1; **(d)** Ad-2 E1A + T24 Ha-*ras* 1; **(e)** *pmt;* **(f)** Ad-2 E1A + *pmt;* **(g)** Ad-2 E1B; **(h)** Ad-2 E1A + Ad-2 E1B. The duration of each assay was 28 days except for **(d)**, which was 18 days. [From Ruley (38).]

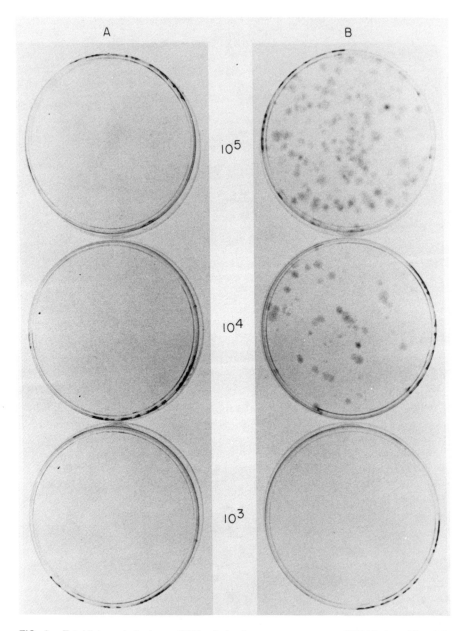

FIG. 2. Establishment of primary BRK cells by the v-*myc* oncogene of MC29 virus. The ability of the v-*myc* oncogene to promote establishment was demonstrated by the outgrowth of colonies after transfected cells were plated in dilute culture. Cell cultures transfected with rat carrier DNA **(A)** or carrier plus pv-*myc* plasmid DNA **(B)** were trypsinized 3 weeks posttransfection and replated at 10^5, 10^4, and 10^3 cells per 60-mm dish. The plates were fixed and stained with Giemsa after 3 weeks. [From Ruley et al. (40).]

transfected BRK cells or BRK cells transfected by *ras* oncogenes failed altogether to form colonies.

The list of oncogenes that enable activated *ras* genes to transform primary rodent cells has grown to include p53 (14,18,34), N-*myc* (42,56), and *myb* [cited in Parada et al. (34)]; p53 facilitated establishment of primary rat chondracytes, and it seems likely that, when tested, N-*myc* and *myb* will possess similar establishment functions. In a similar vein, susceptibility of hamster embryo cells to transformation by *ras* oncogenes coincided with *in vitro* establishment induced by chemical carcinogens (32). Together, these studies further suggested that oncogenic transformation of certain primary rodent cells requires at least two complementing activities that separately promote establishment and acquisition of tumorigenic phenotypes.

ANALYSIS OF E1A TRANSFORMING FUNCTIONS

Coding sequences for three related proteins are generated by differential splicing of adenovirus early-region 1A transcripts during lytic infection. Proteins containing 289 and 243 amino acids are encoded by 13S and 12s mRNAs, respectively. Splicing maintains the reading frames of both mRNAs; therefore the 289 and 243 amino acid proteins differ only by 46 internal amino acids. A third splice generates 9S transcripts, which are most abundant late during lytic infection but have not been detected in transformed cells (52).

For further analysis of E1A transforming functions, plasmids expressing mutant E1A genes were transfected into primary BRK cells alone or together with either T24 Ha-*ras* or *pmt* (59). Transcription and translation products encoded by mutant E1A genes are summarized in Fig. 3. MT13S, MTEB12S, and MTEB9S individually express E1A 13S, 12S, and 9S mRNAs, respectively; pHrI and pHrA contain region 1A genes derived from Ad5 HrI and Hr440 (HrA) adenovirus-5 host range mutants; and dl343 deletes two nucleotides within E1A, resulting in the synthesis of a truncated peptide derived from the amino terminus.

These studies assessed whether E1A plasmids could facilitate *in vitro* establishment or collaborate with T24 Ha-*ras* or *pmt* genes in primary cell transformation. Results summarized in Table 1 further demonstrated that activities that collaborate with T24 Ha-*ras* were linked to activities that facilitate *in vitro* establishment. Moreover, amino terminal sequences common to the 289 and 243 amino acid proteins expressed both transforming functions.

Genes that facilitate establishment, however, do not induce identical phenotypes when transfected individually or together with other oncogenes. This is illustrated by morphological phenotypes of BRK cells established by E1A or transformed by E1A in collaboration with T24 Ha-*ras* or *pmt* (Fig. 4). Moreover, as indicated in Table 2, BRK cells transformed with *hrl* and T24 Ha-*ras* were not tumorigenic in syngenic rats. Other studies have noted similar differences. In particular, early-

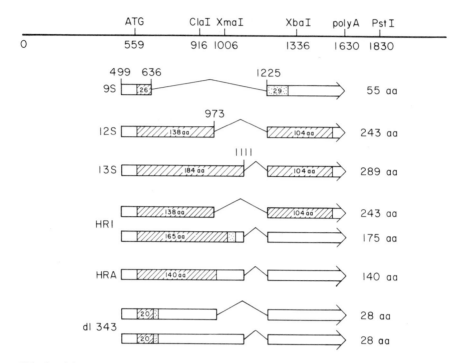

FIG. 3. Adenovirus E1A transcription and translation products. Adenovirus early-region 1A transcripts*(open arrows)* and protein coding sequences *(hatched or stippled regions)* are represented schematically. *Hatched areas* correspond to the reading frame which encodes the 289 and 243 amino acid E1A proteins; *stippled areas* represent alternative translational reading frames; pMTEB9S encodes the E1A 9S mRNA and 55 amino acid protein; pMTEB12S encodes the E1A 12S mRNA and 243 amino acid protein; pMT13S encodes the E1A 13S mRNA and 289 amino acid protein; pHr1 transcripts are spliced to 12S and 13S mRNAs, and express a truncated form of the 289 amino acid protein; pHrA transcripts are spliced to the 13s mRNA, which encodes a truncated polypeptide of 140 amino acids; d1343 synthesizes the 12S and 13S mRNAs and encodes a truncated polypeptide containing 28 amino acids of which eight amino acids are out of frame. [From Zerler et al. (59).]

passage rat embryo cells transformed by T24 Ha-*ras* and E1A and *plt* formed progressively growing tumors in nude mice, whereas transformants generated by T24 Ha-*ras* and *myc* or p53 did not (14,24,34,38). The significance of these phenotypic differences is unknown; however, in one study, tumorigenicity of *ras/myc* cotransformants appeared to require additional genetic alterations (33).

Not all plasmids separately expressing establishment and transforming activities collaborate to transform primary cells. Thus, as indicated in Table 1, E1A mutant *hrA* failed to collaborate with *pmt* to transform primary BRK cells; *hrA* thus resembles *plt,* which did not enable *pmt* to transform primary REF (35). Perhaps in a similar vein, E1B failed to transform morphologically cells of an established line (51). Therefore activities that promote *in vitro* establishment, while perhaps neces-

TABLE 1. *Transforming activities of E1A and v-myc genes[a]*

Gene	Facilitates establishment of primary BRK cells	Collaboration to induce transformed foci	
		With T24 Ha-*ras*	With *pmt*
MTE1A	+	+	+
MT13S	+	+	+
MTEB12S	+	+	+
MTEB9S	−	−	−
HrI	+	+	+
HrA	+[b]	+	−
d1343	−	−	−
v-*myc*	+	+	No data

[a]Plasmids expressing wild-type and mutant adenovirus early-region transcription units or v-*myc* genes were introduced into primary BRK cells individually and together with plasmids expressing the T24 Ha-*ras* and polyoma virus middle T antigen *(pmt)* genes. The ability of E1A and v-*myc* to facilitate establishment of primary BRK cells and to collaborate with T24 Ha-*ras* and *pmt* to induce transformed foci is indicated (+).
[b]Establishment activities were low compared with other E1A plasmids.

sary, are not sufficient for transformation by *pmt* and E1B genes. As discussed in the next section, *in vitro* establishment also does not enable activated *ras* oncogenes to transform cells of the REF52 rat line.

The biochemical functions of E1A proteins are unknown; however, several biological activities are induced by E1A proteins. In particular, adenovirus genes are coordinately regulated during lytic infection, and efficient transcription of viral early-region genes requires activities supplied by the 289 protein (6,19). Both E1A proteins can influence expression of certain nonviral genes, either resident within the genome or carried on transfected plasmids. However, the 243 protein is active only with a subset of genes affected by the 289 protein (1,8,16, 20,27,41,46,49,54). Finally, both E1A proteins enhance adenovirus replication in quiescent cells (29) and stimulate cellular DNA synthesis (5,44); however, only the 289 protein stimulates measureable cell-cycle progression (5).

Whether these biological activities contribute to transformation is presently unknown, but together they implicate transcription and DNA replication as targets of E1A functions. Transcriptional activities of E1A are particularly interesting, since associations between transcriptional activation and transformation have been made for other oncogene proteins (23); however, experimental evidence linking transcriptional effects and transformation is inconclusive. On the one hand, amino terminal sequences shared by the 289 and 243 proteins lack activities of the 289 protein that activate viral gene expression (59). On the other hand, transcription and transformation phenotypes could result from different thresholds of a single activ-

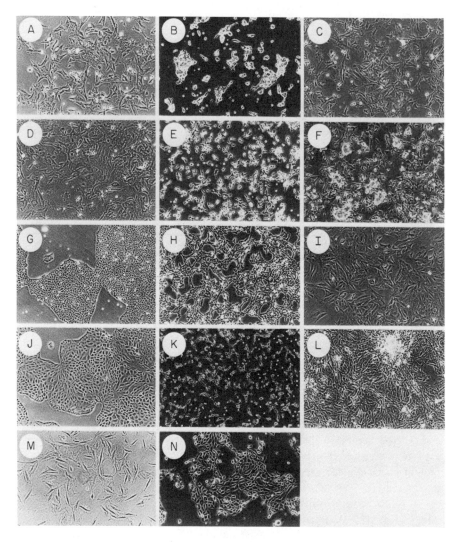

FIG. 4. Established and transformed BRK cell clones. Primary BRK cells were established by transfecting E1A genes alone or were transformed by cotransfecting E1A and either T24 Ha-*ras* or polyoma virus middle T antigen *(pmt):* **(A)** MTE1A; **(B)** MTE1A + T24 Ha-*ras*; **(C)** MTE1A + Py middle T; **(D),** MT13S; **(E)** MT13S + T24 Ha-*ras*; **(F)** pMT13S + *pmt;* **(G)** MTEB12S; **(H)** MTEB12S + T24 Ha-*ras* **(I),** MTEB12S + *pmt;* **(J)** *hrl;* **(K)** *hrl* + T24 Ha-*ras*; **(L)** *hrl* + *pmt;* **(M)** *hrA;* **(N)** *hrA* + T24 Ha-*ras*. Clones derived from transformed foci **(B, C, E, F, H, I, K, L, N)** were photographed after approximately 30 cell doublings. Established clones derived following transfection of E1A plasmids alone **(A, D, G, J, M)** were photographed after 40–60 doublings. All photomicrographs were taken using an 10× objective and were printed at identical magnifications. [From Zerler et al. (59).]

TABLE 2. *Tumorigenicity of BRK cell lines established by E1A and v-myc genes or transformed by E1A and v-myc in collaboration with T24 Ha-ras*[a]

Gene	Established lines	T24 Ha-*ras* cotransformant
MTE1A	−	+
MT13S	−	+
MTEB12S	−	+
Hrl	−	−
HrA	−	+
v-*myc*	−	+

[a]Tumorigenicity was monitored following subcutaneous injection of 10^6 cells into 14-day-old syngeneic rats. Three transformed lines generated with E1A or *myc* genes were injected into each of four animals. Tumorigenic (+) cotransformants gave rise to lethal tumors within 4 weeks in at least half of the injected animals; whereas none of the nontumorigenic (−) lines induced visible tumors by 12 weeks.

ity rather than from genetically separatable biochemical activities. Moreover, viral and cellular genes may differ in their responses to E1A.

MULTISTEP TRANSFORMATION OF REF52 CELLS

REF52 is an established line derived from Fisher rat embryo cells (28). Microinjection and DNA transfection studies demonstrated that activated *ras* genes transform REF52 cells only at low frequencies, and E1A efficiently enables *ras* oncogenes to transform REF52 to a tumorigenic phenotype (15,39). Oncogenes were introduced into REF52 cells by cotransfecting genes encoding the bacterial enzymes, aminoglycoside transferase *(aph)* or guanine phosphoribosyl transferase *(gpt)* as selectable markers. These genes, under the control of eukaryotic transcription and RNA processing signals, enable transfected cells to grow in media containing the neomycin analogue, G418 (SV*aph*) or to use xanthine as a precursor in guanine nucleotide biosynthesis (SV*gpt*).

As shown in Table 3, only a small percentage of G418-resistant colonies generated with cotransfected *ras* oncogenes were morphologically transformed; the vast majority were morphologically indistinguishable from parental REF52 cells. By contrast, a high proportion of G418-resistant colonies generated with cotransfected *ras* and E1A genes were morphologically transformed. Cells transfected by E1A were morphologically altered but were not transformed, as indicated by failure to form tumors in nude mice or to grow in semisolid media. Phase-contrast photomicrographs of G418-resistant colonies generated by transfecting SV*aph,* SV*aph*

TABLE 3. *E1A and T24 Ha-*ras *oncogenes collaborate to transform REF52 cells*[a]

Gene	G418-resistant colonies/10^6 cells	Percent morphologically transformed
aph	400	0
T24aph	300	0.08
E1Aaph	800	0
T24aph + E1Aaph	600	50

[a]Plasmids were transfected onto REF52 cells; transfected cultures were passaged into media containing G418; and colonies resistant to G418 were fixed and stained after 3 weeks. The total number of G418-resistant colonies and the percent of colonies that were morphologically transformed (not including E1A-induced morphologies) are indicated.

linked to E1A, SV*aph* linked to T24 Ha-*ras*, and SV*aph* linked to T24 Ha-*ras*, together with E1A are shown in Fig. 5.

Failure of T24 Ha-*ras* to transform REF52 cells did not result from an absence of gene expression, since the majority of G418-resistant lines expressed *ras* p21 species diagnostic of the T24 Ha-*ras* oncogene (15). However, T24 Ha-*ras* p21 levels were characteristically much lower in cell lines derived by transfecting T24 Ha-*ras* alone (termed T24REF) than in lines transformed by a combination of T24 Ha-*ras* and E1A.

Although expressed at low levels, T24 Ha-*ras* genes in T24REF cells could still participate in transformation, if E1A genes were introduced subsequently (15). For this, E1A was linked to SV*gpt* and transfected into T24REF cells. Among colonies surviving *gpt* selection, greater than 50% were morphologically transformed (Fig. 6). The reciprocal experiment was also successful; thus, REF52 cells initially transfected by E1A*aph* were efficiently transformed by T24 Ha-*ras*. These results indicate that transformation of REF52 cells can occur in a stepwise manner by complementing oncogenes.

As mentioned above, T24 Ha-*ras* transformed REF52 cells at low frequencies in the absence of E1A. The resulting transformants initially grew well when passaged to larger culture vessels; however, by 19 population doublings, growth rates slowed and by 21 doublings, net growth nearly ceased altogether (Fig. 7). Growth arrest was accompanied by severe morphological crisis (Fig. 8a), and more than 90% of the clones were lost prior to 23 population doublings as a result of cell death or displacement by more rapidly growing normal cells.

Although difficulties growing transformants induced by T24 Ha-*ras* alone made further analysis difficult, T24 Ha-*ras* p21 levels were measured in three transformants by means of two-dimensional gel electrophoresis (Fig. 8B). All expressed T24 Ha-*ras* p21 at levels exceeded only by the most abundant cellular proteins. This result indicates that even extremely high levels of T24 Ha-*ras* p21 are unable to induce stable transformation of REF52 cells in the absence of E1A.

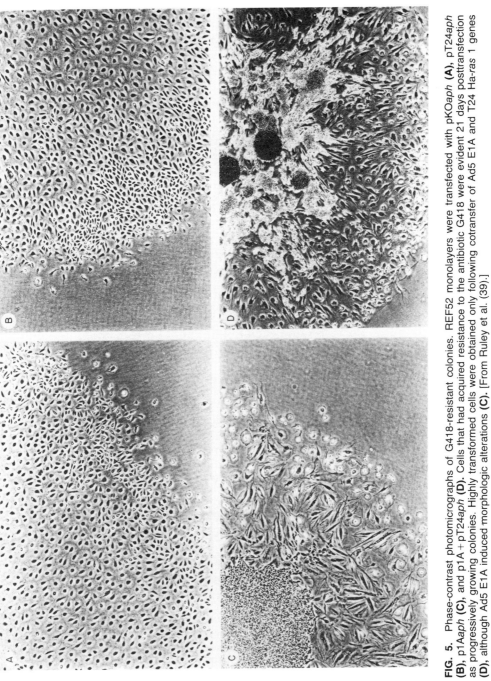

FIG. 5. Phase-contrast photomicrographs of G418-resistant colonies. REF52 monolayers were transfected with pKO*aph* (**A**), pT24*aph* (**B**), p1A*aph* (**C**), and p1A + pT24*aph* (**D**). Cells that had acquired resistance to the antibiotic G418 were evident 21 days posttransfection as progressively growing colonies. Highly transformed cells were obtained only following cotransfer of Ad5 E1A and T24 Ha-*ras* 1 genes (**D**), although Ad5 E1A induced morphologic alterations (**C**). [From Ruley et al. (39).]

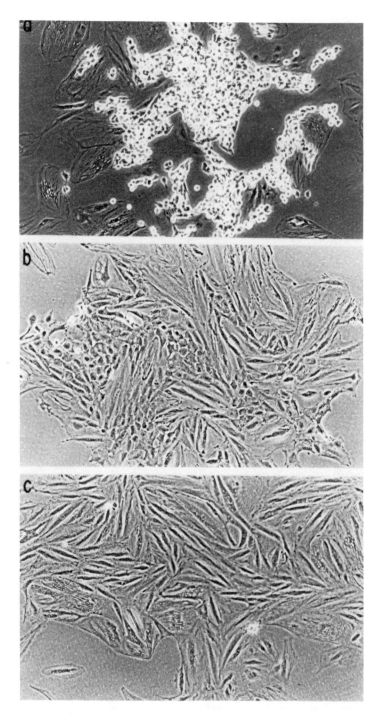

FIG. 6. Stepwise transformation of REF52 cells. Photomicrographs of *gpt* colonies demonstrating that cells which constitutively express T24 Ha-*ras* (clone RN12) are transformed by E1A linked to SV*gpt* **(a)** but not by SV*gpt* alone **(c)**; REF52 cells that do not express T24 Ha-*ras* are not transformed by E1A*gpt* **(b)**.

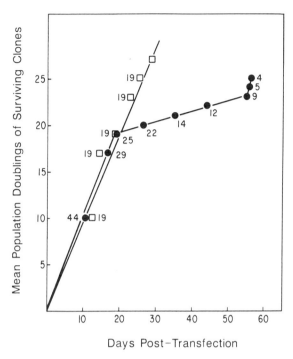

Days Post-Transfection

FIG. 7. Outgrowth of transformed clones. Cells from transformed G418-resistant colonies generated by T24 Ha-*ras* alone [(●) 44 clones] or by activated *ras* genes and E1A [(□) 19 clones] were trypsinized within cloning cylinders and expanded into mass culture. Mean population doublings for surviving clones were estimated when cells were passaged to larger culture vessels. For example, transformed colonies were estimated to contain 10^3 cells (10 population doublings); a confluent 2-cm^2 well, 10^5 cells (17 population doublings); a 35-mm dish, 5×10^5 cells (19 population doublings); a confluent 60-mm dish, 2×10^6 cells (21 population doublings); and a confluent 10-cm dish, 8×10^6 cells (23 population doublings). The number of surviving clones are indicated.

DISCUSSION

Gene-transfer experiments have defined limitations with regard to the ability of individual oncogenes to transform cultured cells. Cells from many established cell lines respond to transfected *ras* and *pmt* genes by morphological transformation and conversion to a tumorigenic phenotype. By contrast, *ras* and *pmt* oncogenes oncogenically transform certain primary rodent cells only at low frequencies unless cotransfected with collaborating genes such as E1A or *myc*. Collaborating genes also promote *in vitro* establishment, whereas neither *ras* nor *pmt* efficiently overturn cellular commitments toward growth arrest and sencescence. These results suggest that oncogenic transformation can require at least two complementing activities that separately enable cultured cells to escape senescence and to acquire tumorigenic phenotypes.

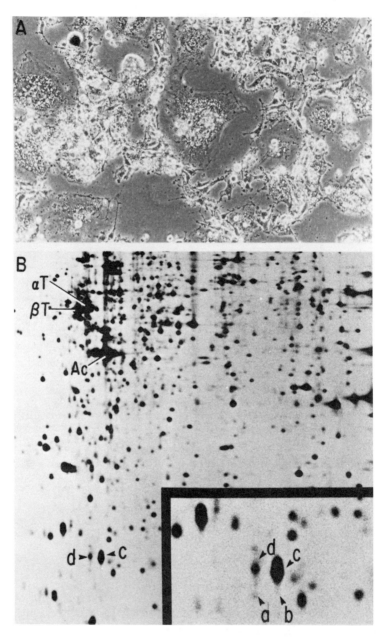

FIG. 8. Morphology and T24 Ha-*ras* expression in REF52 cells transformed by T24 Ha-*ras* in the absence of E1A. **A:** Phase-contrast photomicrographs of transformants induced by T24 Ha-*ras* (clone D12) cells after 21 population doublings. **B:** Two-dimensional gel analysis of [^{35}S]methionine-labeled proteins indicates that T24 Ha-*ras* p21 is overexpressed in unstable transformants (clone D12) induced by T24 Ha-*ras*. Spots *c* and *d* correspond to *p21* proteins encoded by the T24 Ha-*ras* gene; *a* and *b* indicate positions where certain endogenous *p21*'s would be expected to migrate; however, these proteins were not expressed at levels sufficient for detection; αT, βT, and Ac refer to cellular α and β tubulin and actin, respectively. Similar results were obtained with two other unstable transformants induced by T24 Ha-*ras* in the absence of E1A. (R. Franza, *unpublished data*).

Studies with REF52 cells demonstrate that cellular immortality alone does not enable cultured rodent cells to be transformed by *ras* oncogenes. In particular, REF52 cells are refractile to low levels of T24 Ha-*ras* p21 as judged by cell morphology, and even when overexpressed, T24 Ha-*ras* induces morphological crisis and growth arrest rather than stable transformation. Difficulties in transforming primary cells, therefore, need not reflect an inability to superimpose transformed phenotypes over a dominant commitment to senesce.

At a biological level, it is not clear how E1A, a gene concerned with immortalization, enables *ras* oncogenes to transform REF52 cells, but several mechanisms merit discussion. First, *in vitro* establishment may be secondary to other phenotypes induced by E1A. For example, E1A may cause primary cells to proliferate in culture by enhancing responsiveness to serum growth factors. Indeed, genes that facilitate establishment often reduce serum requirements of transfected cells (22,30,35). Moreover, susceptibility of cultured cells toward oncogenic transformation correlates with initial growth factor responsiveness (21). REF52, although established, may be unable to synthesize or respond to activities induced by serum growth factors with efficiencies necessary for transformation by activated *ras* genes. Considering that *ras* may transduce signals from growth factor receptors, E1A may also confer responsiveness to *ras* effector functions.

Second, it is possible that activated *ras* p21 induces a senescent state in REF52 cells if expressed at levels necessary for transformation. E1A may therefore enable *ras* oncogenes to transform both primary cells and REF52 by similar mechanisms. Support for this model is indirect; nevertheless, REF52 cells expressing high *ras* p21 levels experience growth crisis reminiscent of cultured primary cells (15). Whether more physiological p21 levels also induce growth arrest is not known, since T24REF cells invariably express low levels of T24 Ha-*ras* p21. This model implies that *in vitro* immortality is not a dominant phenotype and that *ras* oncogenes can adversely influence maintenance of phenotypic immortality.

Further experiments should clarify biological mechanisms whereby E1A and *ras* collaborate in transformation; however, it should be noted that *ras* and *myc* genes may fail to convert normal cells to a tumorigenic phenotype *in vivo* as well as *in vitro*. For example, activated *ras* genes have been detected in benign skin papillomas, and hormonal stimulation appears to enable carcinogen-activated Ha-*ras* genes to participate in mammary carcinogenesis (3,58). Similarly, *myc* expression is not sufficient to induce either mammary carcinomas in transgenic mice (45) or malignant bursal tumors in chickens (2,31). Therefore, complementations observed between certain oncogenes *in vitro* appear to have some relevance with regard to multistep carcinogenesis *in vivo*. It remains to be determined whether phenotypes induced by individual oncogenes correspond to specific steps in carcinogenesis. Although certain oncogenes appear associated with particular disease stages, such as amplification of N-*myc* in advanced neuroblastoma (10), these may be the exception rather than the rule.

Failure to correlate disease phenotypes with specific oncogenes would not be surprising, since individual oncogenes can induce multiple phenotypes *in vitro*, depending on the target cell and levels of oncogene expression. For example, transcriptional enhancers and coselection in G418 enable *ras* oncogenes to transform early-passage rodent cells without collaborating genes (43); *myc* and E1A induce transformed foci in some cell types but not on others (22,26,43). *Ras* can also promote proliferation and *in vitro* establishment of primary cells (37,43) and differentiation and growth arrest in rat pheochromocytoma cells (4); *myc* and p53 both oncogenically transform certain established cells while inducing only minimal changes in cell morphology (13,22), and retroviral *myc* genes can convert rat embryo cells to a tumorigenic state (55). Finally, synergistic actions of chemical carcinogens and tumor promoters apparently do not involve consistent contributions by individual oncogenes. Thus, initiating events in mouse keratinocytes have been linked to *ras* activation (3,57), whereas initiation in rodent embryo cells has been associated with *myc, plt,* and *in vitro* establishment (12).

Clearly, cell phenotypes do not reflect unique attributes conferred on cells by the activities of individual oncognes. There are many potential reasons for this, but space permits only a brief discussion of these issues. First, oncogenes can collaborate with activities expressed in different target cells to generate multiple phenotypes. This was demonstrated by the fact that T24REF and REF52 have similar morphologies; yet, E1A transforms T24REF because of endogenous T24 Ha-*ras* expression (15). Second, oncogene proteins affect cells at many levels, altering protein modifications and gene expression and eliciting mechanisms to down-regulate cellular responses. Variations in these undoubtedly influence phenotypes induced by introduced oncogenes. Given what we assume are a large number of interacting pathways, it is not surprising that a single oncogene can induce multiple phenotypes in different target cells.

These considerations imply that dominant phenotypes induced by a single oncogene reveal little about underlying metabolic targets or biochemical activities that enable an oncogene to alter cell phenotypes. By contrast, complementations require that phenotypes induced by one oncogene be conditional on activities supplies by other oncogenes. In this regard, complementations are concerned less with cell phenotypes than with the implied interactions between biochemical activities. It is possible that some collaborations between oncogenes reflect summations of related activities, as opposed to genetic complementation. Summation might be suspected if a collaborating oncogene only increased the frequency of transformation or if overexpression of one oncogene induced phenotypes similar to those achieved by collaborating oncogenes. It is also important that phenotypes be evaluated in the same cell type. By these criteria, transformations of primary BRK and REF52 cells by *ras* oncogenes require complementing activities supplied by genes such as E1A and *myc*. Complementations of this type have several applications with regard to analyzing oncogene functions.

First, it has been possible to classify certain oncogenes with regard to phenotypes generated in collaboration with other oncogenes. It is interesting that genes such as E1A, *plt, myc, myb,* and p53, which enable *ras* to transform primary cells and facilitate establishment, are similar in other respects. In particular, all encode nuclear proteins, and some share similarities in protein sequence, short half-life, and ability to influence cellular gene expression [reviewed in Bishop (7)]. Similarities shared by early-region genes of DNA tumor viruses and certain oncogenes expressed in human tumor cells may also have implications concerning biochemical functions. Presumably, the virus-encoded activities are concerned with creating or maintaining permissive cellular environments for viral DNA replication. The viral genes may mimic or activate analogous activities expressed by cellular protooncogenes.

Potentially important differences distinguish these genes as well. Thus, *myc* and *plt* proteins bind DNA, a property not apparently shared by E1A (7). Moreover, E1A sequences most homologous to *myc* are not required to collaborate with *ras* in primary cell transformation (P. Whyte et al., unpublished data). Finally, as discussed previously, genes that facilitate establishment do not induce indentical phenotypes when introduced into primary cells, either individually or together with other oncogenes.

Second, interactions between oncogenes should contribute to understanding the biochemical functions of each participating oncogene. For example, *ras* p21 shares structural and functional similarities with several guanosine triphosphate-regulated signal transducers (9,11,48). Mutations that activate *ras* may alter levels of cellular signals regulated by *ras* effector functions; thus, E1A may influence whether cells synthesize or respond to these signals. E1A could collaborate with *ras* at many levels, from altering receptor levels to influencing nuclear responses to signals regulated by *ras* effector functions. E1A may also act indirectly, for example, by altering cell gene expression; however, even if E1A acts indirectly, oncogene complementations should allow biologically significant genes regulated by E1A to be identified.

Third, cells transformed by two or more complementing oncogenes can be used to analyze biochemical functions of each participating oncogene in the absence of secondary changes brought about by transformation. Thus, signals regulated by *ras* may be easier to analyze in untransformed T24REF than in transformed cells, particularly if transformation down-regulates *ras* functions or conceals *ras* signals among secondary changes. In addition, untransformed cells expressing one of two complementing oncogenes can be manipulated in ways that are not possible with transformed cells. For example, T24REF cells growth arrest in low serum, and this should allow growth factor requirements of REF52 and REF52 cells expressing activated *ras* genes to be compared. Differences may reveal associations between *ras* proteins and specific growth factor receptors. Finally, cells refractile to one oncogene may prove useful as recipients in gene-transfer experiments by allowing genes that express complementing activities to be detected and cloned.

ACKNOWLEDGMENTS

I wish to thank Kazuo Maruyama, Bob Franza, Terri Grodzicker, John Moomaw, Brad Zerler, and Betty Moran, who have all collaborated on the studies described here. This work was supported by grants from the National Cancer Institute, the Robertson Research Fund, and the Whitaker Health Sciences Fund. H.E.R. is a scholar of the Rita Allen Foundation.

REFERENCES

1. Allan, M., Zhu, J.-D., Montague, P., and Paul, J. (1984): Differential response of multiple ε-globin cap sites to *cis-* and *trans*-acting controls. *Cell,* 38:399–407.
2. Baba, T.W., and Humphries, E.H. (1985): Formation of a transformed follicle is necessary but not sufficient for development of an avian leukosis virus-induced lymphoma. *Proc. Natl. Acad. Sci. U.S.A.,* 82:213–216.
3. Balmain, A., Ramsden, M., Bowden, G.T., and Smith, J. (1984): Activation of the mouse cellular Harvey-*ras* gene in chemically induced benign skin papillomas. *Nature,* 307:658–660.
4. Bar-Sagi, D., and Feramisco, J.R. (1985): Microinjection of the *ras* oncogene protein into PC12 cells induces morphological differentiation. *Cell,* 42:841–848.
5. Bellett, A.J.D., Li, P., David, E.T., Macky, E.J., Braithwaite, A.W., and Cutt, J.R. (1985): Control functions of adenovirus transformation region E1A gene products in rat and human cells. *Mol. Cell. Biol.,* 5:1933–1939.
6. Berk, A.J., Lee, F., Harrison, T., Williams, J., and Sharp, P.A. (1979): Pre-early adenovirus 5 gene product regulates synthesis of early viral messenger RNAs. *Cell,* 17:935–944.
7. Bishop, J.M. (1985): Viral oncogenes. *Cell,* 42:23–38.
8. Borelli, E., Hen, R., and Chambon, P. (1984): Adenovirus-2 E1A products repress enhancer-induced stimulation of transcription. *Nature,* 312:608–612.
9. Bourne, H.R. (1985): Yeast *ras* and Tweedledee's logic. *Nature,* 317:16–17.
10. Brodeur, G.M., Seeger, R.C., Schwab, M., Varmus, H.E., and Bishop, J.M. (1984): Amplification of N-*myc* in untreated human neuroblastomas correlates with advanced disease stage. *Science,* 224:1121–1124.
11. Broek, D., Samiy, N., Fasano, O., Fujiyama, A., Tamanoi, F., Northrup, J., and Wigler, M. (1985): Differential activation of yeast adenylate cyclase by wild-type and mutant *ras* proteins. *Cell,* 41:763–769.
12. Connan, G., Rassoulzadegan, M., and Cuzin, F. (1985): Focus formation in rat fibroblasts exposed to a tumor promoter after transfer of polyoma *plt* and *myc* oncogenes. *Nature,* 314:277–279.
13. Eliyahu, D., Michalowitz, D., and Oren, M. (1985): Overproduction of p53 antigen makes established cells highly tumorigenic. *Nature,* 316:158–160.
14. Eliyahu, D., Raz, A., Gruss, P., Givol, D., and Oren, M. (1984): Participation of p53 cellular tumor antigen in transformation of normal embryonic cells. *Nature,* 312:646–649.
15. Franza, B.R., Maruyama, K., Garrels, J.I., and Ruley, H.E. (1986): *In vitro* establishment is not a sufficient prerequisite for transformation by activated *ras* oncogenes. *Cell,* 44:409–419.
16. Green, M.R., Triesman, R., and Maniatis, T. (1983): Transcriptional activation of cloned human β-globin genes by viral immediate early gene products. *Cell,* 35:137–148.
17. Houweling, A., van der Elsen, P.J., and van den Eb, A.J. (1980): Partial transformation of primary rat cells by the leftmost 4.5% fragment of adenovirus 5 DNA. *Virology,* 105:537–550.
18. Jenkins, J.R., Rudge, K., and Currie, G.A. (1984): Cellular immortalization by a cDNA clone encoding the transformation-associated phosphoprotein p53. *Nature,* 312:651–654.
19. Jones, N., and Shenk, T. (1979): An adenovirus type 5 early gene function regulates expression of other early viral genes. *Proc. Natl. Acad. Sci. U.S.A.,* 76:3665–3669.
20. Kao, H.-T., and Nevins, J.R. (1983): Transcriptional activation and subsequent control of the human heat shock gene during adenovirus infection. *Mol. Cell. Biol.,* 3:2058–2065.
21. Kaplan, P.L., and Ozannne, B. (1983): Cellular responsiveness to growth factors correlates with a cell's ability to express the transformed phenotype. *Cell,* 33:931–938.
22. Keath, E.J., Caimi, P.G., and Cole, M.D. (1984): Fibroblast lines expressing activated c-*myc* oncogenes are tumorigenic in nude mice and syngeneic animals. *Cell,* 39:339–348.
23. Kingston, R.E., Baldwin, A.S., and Sharp, P.A. (1985): Transcription control by oncogenes. *Cell,* 41:3–5.
24. Land, H., Parada, L.F., and Weinberg, R.A. (1983): Tumorigenic conversion of primary embryo fibroblasts requires at least two cooperating oncogenes. *Nature,* 304:596–602.
25. Land, H., Parada, L.F., and Weinberg, R.A. (1983): Cellular oncogenes and multistep carcinogenesis. *Science,* 222:771–778.
26. Lautenberger, J.A., Schultz, R.A., Garon, C.F., Tsichlis, P.N., and Papas, T.S. (1981): Molecular cloning of avian myelocytomatosis virus *(MC29)* transforming sequences. *Proc. Natl. Acad. Sci. U.S.A.,* 78:1518–1522.

27. Leff, T., Elkaim, R., Goding, C.R., Jalinot, P., Sassone-Corsi, P., Perricaudet, M., Kodinger, C., and Chambon, P. (1984): Individual products of the adenovirus 12S and 13S E1A mRNAs stimulate viral EIIA and EIII expression at the transcriptional level. *Proc. Natl. Acad. Sci. U.S.A.,* 81:4381–4385.

28. Logan, J., Nicolaus, J.C., Topp, W.C., Giarad, M., Shenk, T., and Levine, A.J. (1981): Transformation by adenovirus early-region 2A temperature sensitive mutants and their revertants. *Virology,* 115:419–422.

29. Montell, C., Fisher, E.F., Carruthers, M.H., and Berk, A.J. (1984): Complete transformation by adenovirus 2 requires both E1A proteins. *Cell,* 36:951–961.

30. Mougneau, E., Lemieux, L., Rassoulzadegan, M., and Cuzin, F. (1984): Biological activities of v-*myc* and rearranged c-*myc* oncogenes in rat fibroblast cells in culture. *Proc. Natl. Acad. Sci. U.S.A.,* 81:5758–5762.

31. Neiman, P., Wolf, C., Enrietto, P.J., and Cooper, G.M. (1985): A retroviral *myc* gene induces preneoplastic transformation of lymphocytes in a bursal transplantation assay. *Proc. Natl. Acad. Sci. U.S.A.,* 82:222–226.

32. Newbold, R.F., and Overell, R.N. (1983): Fibroblast immortality is a prerequisite for transformation by the EJ cHa-*ras* oncogene. *Nature,* 304:648–651.

33. Oshimura, M., Gilmer, T.M., and Barrett, J.C. (1985): Nonrandom loss of chromosome 15 in Syrian hamster tumors induced by v-Ha-*ras* plus v-*myc* oncogenes. *Nature,* 316:636–639.

34. Parada, L.F., Land, H., Weinberg, R.A., Wolf, D., and Rotter, V. (1984): Cooperation between gene-encoding *p53* tumour antigen and *ras* in cellular transformation. *Nature,* 312:649–651.

35. Rassoulzadegan, M., Cowie, A., Carr, A., Glaichenhaus, N., Kamen, R., and Cuzin, F. (1982): The roles of individual polyoma virus early proteins in oncogenic transformation. *Nature,* 300:713–718.

36. Rassoulzadegan, M., Naghashfar, Z., Cowie, A., Carr, A., Grisoni, M., Kamen, R., and Cuzin, F. (1983): Expression of the large T protein of polyoma virus promotes the establishment in culture of "normal" fibroblast cell lines. *Proc. Natl. Acad. Sci. U.S.A.,* 80:4354–4358.

37. Rein, A., Keller, J., Schultz, A.M., Holmes, K.L., Medicus, R., and Ihle, J.N. (1985): Infection of immune mast cells by Harvey sarcoma virus: Immortalization without loss of requirement for interleukin-3. *Mol. Cell. Biol.,* 5:2257–2264.

38. Ruley, H.E. (1983): Adenovirus early region 1A enables viral and cellular transforming genes to transform primary cells in culture. *Nature,* 304:602–606.

39. Ruley, H. E., Moomaw, J., Chang, C., Garrels, J.I., Furth, M., and Franza, R.B. (1985): Multistep transformation of an established cell line by the adenovirus E1A and T24 Ha-*ras* 1 gene. In: *Cancer Cells 3,* Vol. 3, edited by J. Feramisco, B. Ozanne, and L. Stiles, pp. 257–264. Cold Spring Harbor Laboratory, Cold Spring Harbor, New York.

40. Ruley, H.E., Moomaw, J.F., and Maruyama, K. (1984): Avian myelocytomatosis virus *myc* and adenovirus early region 1A promote the *in vitro* establishment of cultured primary cells. In: *Cancer Cells,* Vol. 2: *Oncogenes and Viral Genes,* edited by G.F. Vande Woude, A.J. Levine, W.C. Topp, and Watson, J.D., pp. 481–486. Cold Spring Harbor Laboratory, Cold Spring Harbor, New York.

41. Schrier, P.I., Bernards, R., Vaesson, R.T.M.J., Houweling, A., and van der Eb, A.J. (1983): Expression of class I major histocompatibility antigens switched off by highly oncogenic adenovirus 12 in transformed rat cells. *Nature,* 305:771–775.

42. Schwab, M., Varmus, H.E., and Bishop, J.M. (1985): Human N-*myc* gene contributes to neoplastic transformation of mammalian cells in culture. *Nature,* 316:160–162.

43. Spandidos, D.A., and Wilkie, N.M. (1984): Malignant transformation of early-passage rodent cells by a single mutated human oncogene. *Nature,* 310:469–475.

44. Spindler, K.R., Eng, C.Y., and Berk, A.J. (1985): An adenovirus early-region 1A protein is required for maximal viral DNA replication in growth-arrested human cells. *J. Virol.,* 53:742–750.

45. Stewart, T.A., Pattengale, P.K., and Leder, P. (1984): Spontaneous mammary adenocarcinomas in transgenic mice that carry and express MTV/*myc* fusion genes. *Cell,* 38:627–637.

46. Svensson, C., and Akusjarvi, G. (1984): Adenovirus 2 early-region 1A stimulates expression of both viral and cellular genes. *EMBO J.,* 3:789–794.

47. Thomassen, D.G., Gilmer, T.M., Annab, L.A., and Barrett, J.C. (1985): Evidence for multiple steps in neoplastic transformation of normal and preneoplastic Syrian hamster embryo cells following transfection with Harvey murine sarcoma virus oncogenes (v-Ha-*ras*). *Cancer Res.,* 45:726–732.

48. Toda, T., Uno, I., Ishikawa, T., Powers, S., Katoaka, T., Broak, D., Cameron, S., Broach, J., Matsumoto, K., and Wigler, M. (1985): In yeast, *ras* proteins are controlling elements of adenylate cyclase. *Cell,* 40:27–36.

49. Triesman, R., Green, M.R., and Maniatis, T. (1983): *Cis* and *Trans*-activation of globin transcription in transient assays. *Proc. Natl. Acad. Sci. U.S.A.,* 80:7428–7432.

50. Triesman, R., Novak, U., Favalovo, J., and Kamen, R. (1981): Transformation of rat cells by an altered polyoma virus genome expressing only the middle T protein. *Nature,* 292:595–600.

51. Van den Elsen, P., Houweling, A., and ven der Eb, A. (1983): Expression of region E1b of human adenoviruses in the absence of region E1a is not sufficient for complete transformation. *Virology,* 128:377–390.

52. van der Eb, A.J., and Bernards, R. (1984): Transformation and oncogenecity by adenoviruses. *Curr. Top. Microbiol. Immunol.,* 110:23–51.

53. Varmus, H.E. (1984): The molecular genetics of cellular oncogenes. *Annu. Rev. Genet.,* 18:553–612.

54. Velcich, A., and Ziff, E. (1985): Adenovirus E1A proteins repress transcription from the *SV40* early promoter. *Cell,* 40:705–716.

55. Vennstrom, B., Kahn, P., Adkins, B., Enrietto, P., Hayman, M.J., Graf, T., and Luciw, P. (1984): Transformation of mammalian fibroblasts and macrophages *in vitro* by a murine retrovirus encoding an avian v-*myc* oncogene. *EMBO J.,* 3:3223–3229.

56. Yancopoulos, G.D., Nisen, P.D., Tesfaye, A., Kohl, N.E., Goldfarb, G.P., and Alt, F.W. (1985): N-*myc* can cooperate with *ras* to transform normal cells in culture. *Proc. Natl. Acad. Sci. U.S.A.,* 82:5455–5459.

57. Yuspa, S.H., Kilkenny, A.E., Stanley, J., and Lichti, U. (1985): Keratinocytes blocked in phorbol ester-responsive early stage of terminal differentiation by sarcoma viruses. *Nature,* 314:459–462.

58. Zarbl, H., Sukumar, S., Arthur, A.V., Martin-Zanca, D., and Barbacid, M. (1985): Direct mutagenesis of Ha-*ras*-1 oncogenes by *N*-nitroso-*N*-methylurea during initiation of mammary carcinogenesis in rats. *Nature,* 315:382–385.

59. Zerler, B., Moran, B., Maruyama, K., Moomaw, J., Grodzicker, T., and Ruley, H.E. (1986): Analysis of E1A coding sequences which enable *ras* and *pmt* oncogenes to transform cultured primary cells. *Mol. Cell. Biol.,* 6:887–899.

Advances in Viral Oncology, Volume 6, edited by
George Klein. Raven Press, New York © 1987.

Stepwise Transformation and Cooperative Interactions Involving Oncogenes of DNA Tumor Viruses

F. Cuzin and G. Meneguzzi

*Laboratoire de Génétique Moléculaire des Papovavirus
(INSERM U 273), Centre de Biochimie,
Université de Nice, 06034 Nice, France*

Most oncogenic DNA viruses use more than one gene to transform cells. This peculiarity, originally established for polyomaviruses and adenoviruses (26,93,95,121), and recently suggested also for herpesviruses and papillomaviruses (50,57,108,128), is associated with one of the important differences between the DNA and RNA oncogenic viruses. The transforming genomes of retroviruses [see Graf and Stéhelin (48) for review] are completely defective and as such are not maintained in nature. It is not clear what advantage, if any, is conferred on the virus by its ability to recombine with proto-oncogenes and thereby transform cells, but this event clearly results in the extinction of both the host cell and the viral lineage.

By contrast, DNA viruses have developed cell transformation as a way of propagating complete genomes by vertical transmission. Evolution of their transforming genes could therefore take place, leading to the complex arrangements of specialized functions intricated with those needed for horizontal propagation, which were described by Benjamin (3) as "oncogenes with a purpose." These pleiotropic gene complexes became adapted to either a unique target cell (most papillomaviruses) or a wide spectrum of cell types (polyomaviruses). This process has also led to extensive evolutionary divergence, to the point where the viral oncogenes no longer showed a significant degree of homology with cellular DNA sequences. Studies on retroviruses were essential for the structural analysis of cellular oncogenes and their protein products. DNA tumor viruses, however, because of this fine adjustment to the most essential regulations of their host cells, might now constitute useful tools for the analysis of critical cell controls.

Tumor progression (38,101) is clearly a situation for which we need adequate experimental models. The striking progressiveness of numerous cancers is at variance with the absence of detectable intermediary stages during transformation to a fully tumorigenic state by the unique oncogene of most retroviruses or by cloned cellular oncogenes [see Graf and Stéhelin (48) and Müller and Verma (79) for review]. DNA viruses now appear to participate in a variety of multistage scenarios of oncogenesis, both in nature and in the laboratory. Their association with the progression of human cancers was recognized in several instances, such as Burkitt lymphoma, skin and genital cancers, and liver carcinoma. Several of these clinical aspects are reviewed elsewhere in this Volume; we shall limit this discussion to two experimental cases where multiple viral oncogenes, combinations of viral and cellular genes and of viral oncogenes and chemical promoters were shown to interact along progressive transformation pathways, which may tell us something about the progression of a tumor.

THE MULTIPLE ONCOGENES OF POLYOMAVIRUSES

The small genomes of polyomaviruses are remarkable for the extreme compaction of their genetic information: The same nucleotide sequence may encode several proteins with alternative RNA splicing, allowing the use of two, and sometimes three, reading frames. In addition, distinct domains of a protein may act in different regulatory processes. The two viruses studied most, polyoma and simian virus (SV)40, present extensive physiological similarities and homologies in the primary structures of their proteins. Despite these similarities, their transforming functions differ in many respects, and the two viruses in fact appear to be the prototypes of two distinct subfamilies that share a number of structural and biological features but developed distinct transformation mechanisms.

The "3-T Antigen" Viruses

Until recently, polyoma appeared to be unique because it encodes three early proteins (the large, middle, and small T antigens) and not two, as do SV40 and related viruses [see Hand (53) and Ito (55) for review and Fig. 1]. The family is now likely to increase because a virus isolated from hamster epitheliomas (HaPV) was recently shown to share the same genetic structure (30). Since the pioneer work of Vogt and Dulbecco (123,124), the transforming properties of polyoma have been the subject of intensive studies that established the basic characteristics of its interaction with cells in culture and provided two essential tools for further analysis: a set of transformation-defective mutants (hrt, tsa), which led eventually to the identification of two important oncogenic determinants (middle and large T), and, more recently, a series of genetically engineered viral genes, each encoding only one of the early proteins (24).

Altogether, the three viral proteins appear to constitute an efficient multitarget transforming mechanism. In Table 1 are listed a series of experimental situations that require either one or two or all three. Nothing is known of the functions needed in vivo to transform various differentiated cells. We know that the virus is capable of interacting with different types of cells to induce a wide variety of tumors; an observation that led to its designation as "the virus of many tumours"

TABLE 1. *Polyoma virus proteins required for cell transformation*[a]

Species	Cell type	Conditions	Viral protein(s)	Ref.
Rat/mouse	Embryo fibroblasts	Primary culture (DMEM + 10% FCS)	LT + MT + ST	95–125
Rat/mouse	Established cell lines	Low serum (DMEM + 0.5% CS)	LT + MT	93
		High serum (DMEM + 10% CS)	MT	93–120
Rat	Unknown	*In vivo*	LT + MT or LT + ST	1a

[a](LT, MT, ST): large, middle, and small T proteins; (DMEM): Dulbecco modified Eagle's medium; (FCS): fetal calf serum; (CS) calf serum.

[polyoma; see Stewart (118) for review], and it is tempting to speculate that it may use various combinations of transforming functions, depending on the host cells and the physiological conditions.

The clearest case of tumoral progression is that of fibroblast cells explanted from rodent embryos in midgestation (REF cells). Vogt and Dulbecco (123,124) have suggested that transformation of these most normal cells proceeds through successive stages, with increasingly abnormal morphologies, growth properties, and karyotypes. One such property is that of "immortality," a somewhat dramatic designation for an extended capacity for cell division in a highly artificial environment (calf serum diluted in CO_2-buffered DMEM medium). Among the large variety of other transformation-associated properties that have been described, some were of operational importance because they provided simple selection methods, such as the ability to grow past confluency in suspension or at low serum concentration. The endpoint of the whole process is a cell line that produces fast-growing tumors when injected into syngeneic animals. Although only moderately invasive, these tumors will eventually kill the animal, and metastasis can sometimes be observed.

Expression of a fully transformed phenotype and of tumorigenicity requires the middle T protein. Since the initial discovery of the protein, this requirement has been inferred from a series of converging experimental results, including the transformation-defective phenotype of the large-T-only *hrt* mutants and apparent similarities between the biochemical properties of middle T and of the protein product of the v-*src* oncogene of Rous sarcoma virus [see Ito (55) for review]. The role of middle T, and its limits, was eventually established by Kamen et al. (93,95,120). A modified polyoma genome encoding only this protein has been shown to transform rat fibroblast cells. Unlike the wild-type virus genome, however, it could only transform cells of established lines (Rat-1, FR3T3) and, furthermore, only in high-serum medium. Correlatively, the middle-T-only transformants obtained under these conditions ("MTT lines") appeared to lack the independence from serum factors for growth in culture that is characteristic of polyoma transformants. In low-serum medium, MTT cells did multiply, but they reverted to a normal phenotype, and they could be complemented for anchorage-independent growth and focus formation by transfer of similar constructs encoding only the large T protein (*plt* gene).

Transfer of the gene-encoding-only middle T *(pmt)* did not induce transformation of REF cells. Completion of a first transformation step, dependent on the expression of large T, was required for further transformation of these cells by the *pmt* gene. Cells expressing only large T exhibited a series of new properties (Table 2), the most conspicuous of which was the ability for long-term growth in culture without the concomitant acquisition of tumorigenic properties, as originally observed in 3T3 lines by Todaro and Green (119). Cell lines immortalized by large T did not appear to be "transformed" by several of the classical *in vitro* criteria (focus formation, anchorage independency). A noticeable rate of spontaneous occurrence of fully transformed derivatives was, however, apparent when the lines were propagated in culture for high numbers of generations. In addition, segregation of transformed clones could be induced by a limited exposure to a dose of phorbol ester, which had no effect on REF cells (18). Cells expressing large T thus appear to be "high-risk cells," and one might speculate that this reflects a high frequency of mutation in cellular proto-oncogenes and, more generally, an increased genetic instability induced by the viral protein. Several large-T-only cell lines exhibited aneuploid chromosome numbers, and it will be of interest to measure frequencies of mutation, recombination, and gene amplification in these cells. It may be significant that they exhibit an increased rate of sister chromatid exchange (12a).

Parallel to their susceptibility to spontaneous and chemical transformation, cells expressing large T have been transformed by viral and cellular oncogenes that had no effect on REF cells. This phenomenon, first demonstrated with the polyoma

TABLE 2. *Properties of rat fibroblast cell lines established after transfer of the* plt *gene of polyoma virus (large T protein), of* v-myc *and of rearranged* c-myc *oncogenes*

Similar to normal REF cells
   Low saturation density
   Anchorage dependency
   Flat morphology, organized cytoskeleton
Similar to fully transformed lines
   Continuous growth in culture
   Serum-independent growth
Specific properties
   Reactivity to class II oncogenes (polyoma *pmt;* activated *ras* genes)
   Reactivity to tumor promoters
   Spontaneous transformation
   High sister chromatid exchange frequency

pmt gene (middle T protein), was subsequently extended by Land et al. (62) and by Ruley (104) to other combinations of genes. Cotransfer of polyoma *plt* and of activated *ras* genes led to oncogenic transformation of REF cells. Combinations of *ras* and of rearranged and viral *myc* genes were also efficient, the *myc* oncogenes inducing in rat fibroblast cells all the phenotypic changes previously observed in large-T-only cells (Table 2).

Transformation of REF cells was thus achieved in two steps by successive transfer of two of the polyoma oncogenes, *plt* and *pmt*. Simultaneous transfer of these two genes, however, did not lead to focus formation, unless the third early viral gene, *pst* (small T protein), was also present. Further analysis of this apparent paradox suggested that transformation by *pmt* requires a cellular function that is expressed constitutively in established lines but depends on the small T protein in REF cells. This requirement appears to be specific to middle-T (cotransfer of *plt* and *ras* oncogenes) leading to immediate transformation, whereas focus formation after transfer of *myc* and *pmt* was dependent on the simultaneous presence of *pst* (26).

Although the molecular mechanisms at work are still to a large extent a matter of speculation, what we know of the biochemistry of the two main polyoma effectors, large and middle T, provides us with clues of possible interest.

Large T

Large T is a multifunctional protein localized in the cell chromatin, where it participates in a series of regulatory functions. As the corresponding SV40 protein, it acts in lytically infected cells in the initiation of viral DNA replication (39), and as a pleiotropic transcriptional regulator [repression of the early promotor (17,37) and activation of late transcription (9)], it binds tightly to specific sites [direct repeats of G(purine)GGC pentanucleotides] in the region of the viral genome corresponding to the origin of replication and promoters. Two biochemical properties of the protein were described whose physiological meaning is still unclear: ATPase activity (41) and binding of nucleoside diphosphate (14,16). Distinct functional domains were grossly defined in the protein: Truncated forms corresponding to 40% or more starting from the amino terminus, defective for DNA replication, were fully capable of immortalizing REF cells and of cooperating with the *pmt* and the *ras* oncogenes (62,93,95) but were defective for DNA replication. Deletions within this amino-terminal half of the molecules, however, did not abolish DNA replication (81).

Middle T

Middle T is a membrane-associated protein (55) that can be phosphorylated *in vitro* on tyrosine residues, as previously described, for the product of the v-*src* gene of Rous sarcoma virus. The work of Courtneidge et al. (20,21) and Bolen et al. (7) indicated that tyrosine kinase activity is not a property of middle T itself, but rather of a tightly associated cellular enzyme that has been identified as the product of the c-*src* gene (pp60^{c-src}). Studies using nontransforming mutants of the virus have suggested that formation of the pp60^{c-src}/middle T complex is a necessary event for the occurrence of transformation. Tyrosine kinase activity has been shown to be enhanced in the complex, possibly by changes in the pattern of phosphorylation of the c-*src* kinase. Association with middle T thus appears to be a case of oncogene activation by protein–protein interaction. To what extent the resulting effects are comparable to the mutational events that convert the same c-*src* gene into the v-*src* oncogene [Parker et al. (90) and references therein] remains to be determined.

The "2-T Antigen" Viruses

SV40 is the prototype of a subgroup of polyomaviruses isolated from primates (SV40, BK, JC viruses) that show a complex relationship with their rodent counterparts (polyoma, HaPV). In spite of extended amino acid sequence homologies, especially in the late genes (structural proteins) and in the carboxyterminal part of the early region, which is thought to correspond to the DNA replication functions [see Clertant and Seif (16) for review], the comparison of the complete nucleotide sequence of the polyoma genome with that of SV40 or BK virus (40,115), and the analysis of T antigens by immunoprecipitation [see Ito (55) for review], revealed one major structural difference: The early region of the primate virus encodes only two proteins, which are homologous, respectively, to the polyoma large and small T proteins (Fig. 1). Converging results now suggest that the absence of a middle T protein corresponds to profound differences in the mechanisms developed by the two families of viruses to transform cells. These differences were first detected in the biological properties of the transformed cells. They can now be paralleled by clearly distinct biochemical mechanisms.

Biological Properties of Transformed Cell Lines

Risser and Pollack (99) first described a large variety of phenotypes in SV40-transformed rodent cell lines, ranging from near-normal cells to cell lines with more clearly abnormal growth properties. Most freshly transformed rodent cells exhibit only limited changes and either produce no tumors in syngeneic animals, or, with low efficiency and after long latency periods, produce tumors that in several cases were shown to have lost all SV40 genetic information (29,112). When studied in the same cellular background, this limited transformation potential appeared to be clearly different from the ability of polyoma to induce advanced tumorigenic states (94).

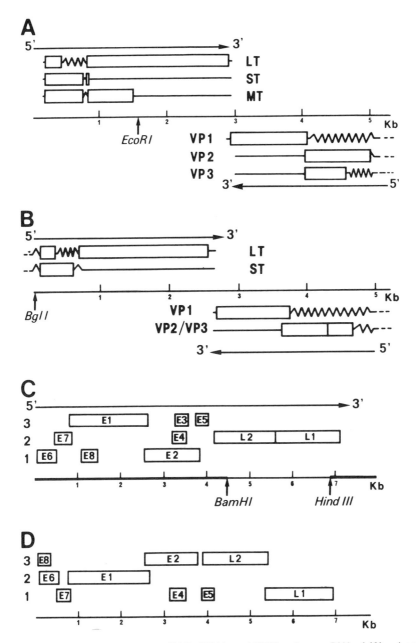

FIG. 1. Genetic maps of polyoma, SV40, BPV1, and HPV1a viruses. DNA of **(A)** polyoma (51) and **(B)** SV40 (11) viruses is linearized at the origin of replication, and the sizes of the early and late messengers are indicated, with the direction of transcription (5′–3′; *arrow*). Coding exons are represented as boxed areas [(LT) large T; (MT) middle T; (ST) small T; (VP1–VP3) late proteins] and spliced introns as staggered segments. DNA of **(C)** BPV1 (13) and **(D)** HPV1a (27) viruses is linearized at the *Hpa*I site, the *arrow* indicating the 5′–3′ direction of BPV1 transcription. Boxed areas correspond to the open reading frames deduced from sequencing data; (E1–E8) early region; (L1, L2) late region.

Intracellular Localization of the Large T Protein

SV40 large T acts in the same regulatory processes as the homologous polyoma protein (initiation of replication, regulation of transcription), and, similarly, most of the protein is found in the nucleus of transformed cells. A small but significant part, however, is present in cell membranes [(31,64); see also Sharma et al. (113) for review], a localization similar to that of middle T in polyoma-transformed cells. One possibility at this stage is to consider that SV40 large T comprises, in addition to domains homologous to those of the polyoma large T protein, sequences that are structurally homologous and functionally equivalent to polyoma middle T. This hypothesis is not quite supported by comparison of amino acid sequences, the homology between polyoma middle T and SV40 large T being limited to a stretch of six acidic residues (40,115). More important, it now appears that the two proteins act on distinct cellular targets, SV40 large T being tightly bound, not to the c-*src* kinase, but to a distinct cellular protein, p53.

The Cellular p53 Tumor Antigen and Its Possible Role in Cell Transformation

A phosphoprotein termed p53 was first discovered being coimmunoprecipitated with SV40 large T in extracts of transformed cells (60,63,68). In fact, elevated levels of p53 were found in a variety of tumor and transformed cells [see Levine et al. (67) for review]. The protein is detectable at a low level in normal cells, and depending on the particular cell line analyzed, the mechanism leading to an increased steady-state level is either transcriptional or post-transcriptional.

Although elevated levels of p53 were not found in all tumor and transformed cells (22), its presence in a large majority of them led to widespread speculation that it might play an important role in cellular growth control. Two series of results are now supporting this view. Studies on cell-cycle control have established that the levels of p53 were low in serum-starved (G0) fibroblasts and increased shortly before DNA synthesis, when cells were stimulated with mitogens (76,96). A role of the protein in the transition from G0 to active growth has been suggested by experiments showing that microinjection of monoclonal antibodies directed against the protein prevented cellular DNA synthesis under these conditions (75). It is not clear, however, that we can infer from these results that the protein plays a role in normal growth control: Unlike the change observed during transition from G0 to G1, no quantitative change was observed when actively growing cells transit from G1 to S to G2 (19). More direct evidence that the protein plays a role in the transformation of REF cells has been found (36,89): Cotransfection of vectors expressing high levels of p53 and of activated *ras* oncogenes led to cell transformation under the conditions previously used for demonstrating cooperation between *myc* and *ras* or between *plt* and *ras* oncogenes (see above).

THE TWO PARADIGMS OF POLYOMAVIRUSES: GENETIC COOPERATION AND STAGE-SPECIFIC ONCOGENES

Polyoma and SV40 offered the original, and still among the clearest, examples of the two now widely popular notions of genetic cooperation in oncogenesis and of stage-specific oncogenes. Although there has been some confusion between these two notions in the past, they are clearly dissociated in some of the work reviewed in this section. In at least two different instances, transformation has been shown to require the *cooperation* of one viral and one cellular gene (polyoma middle T and pp60^{c-src}; SV40 large T and p53). Other such cases are likely to be discovered [for instance, cellular proteins are associated with the small T protein (106,107,127)], the main limitation being in most instances our almost complete ignorance of the biochemistry of the oncogene products. As noted above, these specific associations represent a case of oncogene activation by protein–protein interaction. This does not mean that the cooperating genes participate in a multistep scenario; rather, there is in fact no convincing experimental argument to suggest that SV40 controls more than one step of cell transformation. Cooperation is also not likely to be limited to two partners, one viral and one cellular gene, as exemplified by the adjunctory effect of small T on transformation by middle T (see above). For this reason, the original inference that rearranged *myc* genes and mutated *ras* genes determine two distinct steps of the transformation process, made from the observation that the two genes together transform cells that neither of them could transform separately (62), was an extrapolation from observations in viral systems.

On the other hand, *stepwise transformation* has been demonstrated in the case of polyomavirus by showing that cells that express the large T protein become susceptible to transformation by the *pmt* gene. The intermediary stage (''immortalized'' lines) has been isolated and has been shown to exhibit properties different from both the normal and the fully transformed cells (95). This was eventually also done with *myc* oncogenes (77,105), thus substantiating the hypothesis of a two-step pathway.

Finally, it must be noted that there is no evidence against the notion of a multistep pathway being determined by a single oncogene. Experimental results have suggested in fact that this might be the case for *ras* oncogenes when expressed at very high levels (115a). These gene dosage effects are not unexpected in the case of these most sensitive and central controls of the cell. Several explanations, not exclusive of each other, can be considered. A purely quantitative effect is possible when the same protein acts on distinct targets with different affinities. Alternatively, as exemplified by the polyoma and SV40 large T proteins, distinct domains of a multifunctional protein can act in physiologically distinct pathways. In the case of oncogenes such as *myc* and *plt,* we could consider a third possibility on the basis of our previous conclusion that expression of these genes increases the probability of the cell to progress further toward a highly transformed state, either by activation of other oncogenes, due to an inherent genetic instability, or because it is more responsive to external stimuli. What appears to be a process dependent on one gene only might in fact under these conditions correspond to the induction by this gene of a first stage, followed by additional changes occurring in a significant number of cells. The successive steps may then be difficult to prove, because *in vitro* as well as *in vivo,* selective advantages lead to a rapid spread of the more advanced tumoral phenotypes.

ASSOCIATION OF PAPILLOMAVIRUSES WITH *IN VIVO* TUMOR PROGRESSION AND WITH STEPWISE TRANSFORMATION *IN VITRO*

The oncogenic properties of papillomaviruses formed the basis of one of the very first experimental models of tumoral progression, developed by Rous and his colleagues half a century ago (100,101), and more than 20 years ago, bovine papillomavirus type 1 (BPV1) was shown to transform cells in culture (5,6). Only recently, however, have advances in the technology of genetic determinants permitted research at the molecular level. Results of interest have already appeared, and two observations are especially relevant to our present point of view: (a) the specific association with progressive malignant diseases of the genomes of several human papillomaviruses (HPV), and (b) the original stepwise transformation pathway induced by papillomaviruses in natural and experimental animal systems, including *in vitro* fibroblast cultures. Other areas of interest from the cell biology and molecular biology points of view are the strict dependence of the productive part of the virus cycle on the terminal differentiation of skin keratinocytes and the maintenance in transformed cells of the provirus genome in a plasmidial state [see Lancaster and Olson (61) and Orth (83) for review].

Isolated from epithelial proliferative lesions (warts) in various species including man, the viruses constitute a highly homogeneous group. On the basis of analogies in the structure of the virions, it was initially considered that the Papovaviridae family included two genera, polyomaviruses and papillomaviruses; but these two groups appear now to be distinct in many of their biological and stuctural properties at the molecular level. Virus-induced papillomas have been the subject of extensive clinical and epidemiological studies [see Orth and Favre (85) and Zur Hausen (130) for review], but molecular approaches have been hampered by the lack of a suitable cell culture system. The development of genetic engineering techniques was therefore essential: Molecular cloning in bacteria allowed the isolation of new viral genomes from nonproductive tumors; Southern blot analysis led to the discovery of a number of viral types, and DNA sequencing provided the first elements in our comprehension of their genetic organization [see Danos and Yaniv (28) and Dürst et al. (35) for review]. On the basis of DNA sequence homology, more than 30 different types of human viruses (HPV) and six bovine viruses (BPV) have been identified (Table 3). Despite this variety, papillomaviruses show remarkably constant genetic organization (Fig. 1). All the protein reading frames are located on one strand, indicating unidirectional transcription over the entire genome [approximately 8 kilobases (kb)]. The identification of a subgenomic fragment of BPV1 DNA, sufficient for transformation of rodent cells *in vitro,* the 69% *Bam*HI-*Hin*dIII fragment, and the comparative analysis of the nucleotide sequences of human (HPV1, HPV6b, HPV16), bovine (BPV1), and rabbit viruses [cotton-tail rabbit (or Shope) papillomavirus (CRPV)] have demonstrated in all cases the same arrangements of open reading frames, both in the late region, encoding the capsid proteins, and in the early region, encoding transformation and replication functions. A third region, 1 kb long, contains palindromic sequences, and direct repeats and corresponds to the promoters and origin of replication (13,27,43,69,109,111,125). The number, nature, and functions of the individual viral proteins involved in the oncogenic process remain essentially to be discovered. The recent identification of functions involved in transformation already suggests that more than one viral gene is required, in agreement with the tentative

TABLE 3. *Human and bovine papillomaviruses*

Virus	Type	Initial lesion	Viral types associated with carcinomas
HPV	1–4, 7, 10, 25, 27, 28	Skin warts	10[a]
	3, 5, 8, 9, 12, 14, 15, 17, 19–25	Epidermodysplasia verruciformis	5, 8, 14[a]
	6, 11, 16	Genital warts and papulosis	6, 11[a], 16, 18
	6, 11	Laryngeal papillomas	
	13	Focal epithelial hyperplasia	
	9	Keratoakanthoma	
BPV	1, 2, 5	Fibropapillomas	1[a], 2
	3, 4, 6	Papillomas	4

[a]Low incidence

generalization that opened this chapter (33,80,108,128). Attempts to detect early gene products in cells transformed *in vitro* or in tumor tissue were for a long time unsuccessful, but the first identification of a viral early protein has been recently announced (1a).

Most papillomaviruses show a narrow host range: They infect basal epithelial cells, and productive replication occurs exclusively in differentiating keratinocytes. They produce epithelial or fibroepithelial proliferations of the skin and mucosa. Infectious particles, assembled in the upper layers of the stratum spinosum, spread with scales from the stratum corneum. A subgroup of papillomaviruses, including the most studied member of the group (BPV1) shows, however, a broader host range: These viruses transform dermis fibroblasts [see Lancaster and Olson (61), Orth (83), Pfister (91), and Smith and Campo (114) for review].

Papillomaviruses and Cancer

Although tumors induced by papillomaviruses are generally benign and are capable of only limited growth with frequent spontaneous regression, increasingly striking evidence suggests that some are involved in the etiology of animal and human cancers (Table 3). Since the early analysis by Rous and his colleagues (101) of the frequent conversion to carcinomas of CRPV-induced papillomas, a viral origin has been demonstrated for fibrosarcomas and oesophageal carcinomas in cattle (58), for bovine ocular papilloma (116), and for cutaneous carcinoma in sheep (122). In humans, evolution into squamous neoplasias of benign lesions associated with HPVs, first observed in rare diseases [epidermodysplasia verruciformis (EV), laryngeal papillomatosis], was subsequently extended to the more frequent genital carcinomas [see Glassmann (41), Orth and Favre (85), Pfister (91), and Smith and Campo (114), for review]. Epidermodysplasia verruciformis is a disease usually observed in patients with congenital defects of cell-mediated immunity, which in one third of the cases leads to the development of multiple bowenoid or squamous cell carcinomas. Various HPV viruses have been found to coexist in benign tumors, but only DNA of types 5, 8, and 14 has been found in carcinomas (59,83,87,88,91). An etiological role of papillomaviruses has been independently indicated in juvenile laryngeal papillomatosis, first by histological observations and then by detection of viral antigens and mature particles. HPV6 DNA has been recurrently found in lesions (78), and the genome of a new type (HPV11), has been cloned from a benign papilloma (45). Malignant evolution is enhanced after therapeutic X-ray irradiation but remains a rare event (130). This is not the case for genital cancers, for which epidemiological evidence has suggested the implication of infectious determinants. Papillomaviruses have been added to the list of suspect agents, because HPV DNA was found in biopsies from precancerous lesions of uterine cervix (47,49,129). Although the association of HPV infections with condylomata acuminata was proved in the late 1960s (34,82), a relationship between viral infection and warts of the cervix and vagina was more difficult to establish (2,72,92). It is now clear that the "koilocytotic" cells of flat condylomas contain viral particles. These lesions are clinically indistinguishable from mild cervical dysplasia, and benign forms may coexist with dysplastic and neoplastic epithelium. Spontaneous regression of benign forms is observed in 40% of patients; however, progression to severe dysplasia, to *in situ* carcinoma, or to invasive carcinoma takes place in 10% of cases (117). Since 1.5% of the women present cytological evidence of HPV infection in Papanicolau smears (73,93), efforts have been made to establish a relationship between precancerous lesions with a high risk of malignant evolution and specific pathological parameters (23). Large-scale screening of biopsies from tumoral tissues has revealed the presence of HPV6 and HPV11 DNA sequences, primarily in benign condylomas, whereas HPV16 DNA has been almost exclusively detected in precancerous lesions and invasive carcinomas (36,70). Similar observations have been made on penile precancerous and cancerous lesions (54). DNA sequences of another HPV (type 18) have been found in tumors and in cell lines established from cervical carcinomas (8). In benign lesions, the viral DNA replicates extrachromosomally, but in a fraction of the tumors and tumor-derived cell lines, integration into the host genome has been observed (8,109). Similar findings have been reported for BPV1 and CRPV (10,71,126), but no clear relationship between integration and malignant evolution has so far been established.

Conversely, malignant conversion of papillomas is known to depend on interactions involving both infection with specific viral strains and environmental cofactors, such as tobacco smoke, ultraviolet and X-ray irradiation, genetic background, and chemical carcinogens. Rous and Friedewald (102) have described a synergistic effect of tumor promoters on the malignant evolution of papillomas in the domestic rabbit. More recently, Jarrett et al. (58) have suggested that massive ingestion of a bracken fern induces tumoral progression of cattle papillomatosis.

The presence of viral DNA does not by itself prove a direct role of the viruses in the cancerization process, and efforts have therefore been made to establish *in vitro* model systems in which the transforming potential could be assayed. Ideal cultures to work on are those derived from the natural target cells—those of epithelial basal layers (65). These cells, however, are among the most difficult to maintain *in vitro,* and a number of studies concentrated on the transformation by BPV1 of rodent fibroblast lines [(5,6); see Lancaster and Olson (61) and Pfister (91) for review]. The properties of a series of these rat cell lines were analyzed in our laboratory and compared to those of reference transformants SV40, polyoma, and *ras* oncogenes and to the behavior *in vivo* of the virus-associated papillomas and carcinomas. Artificial as this experimental system may be (genes of a bovine virus expressed in rodent fibroblasts grown in calf serum), it is interesting to note that BPV1 transformants differ from other cell lines in a number of critical properties and follow a reproducible succession of transformation stages similar in some ways to the progression from papilloma to carcinoma.

Stepwise Transformation of Rodent Cell Lines Transfected with BPV1 DNA

BPV1-transformed cell lines were established after transfer into rat FR3T3 cells of purified viral DNA or of pBR322-derived plasmids carrying either the complete viral genome or only its transforming region (4,52). We noted that unlike comparable rodent cells transformed by polyoma, SV40, or cloned *ras* genes, these transformants retained a phenotype close to that of normal fibroblasts. Most noticeably, they kept the flat morphology and the organized cytoskeleton of the normal fibroblast. Moreover, they grew only in the presence of high serum concentrations, exhibited a low plating efficiency in agarose medium, and did not produce plasminogen activator. It was quite striking to observe that in spite of this low level of transformation *in vitro,* these BPV1-transformed cells were highly tumorigenic when injected into syngeneic rats. Tumors developed within 4 to 6 weeks and were considerably more aggressive than polyoma transformants: On subcutaneous inoculation, rapid invasion of the inner organs was observed in all rats, with frequent lung metastasis.

A still more striking discrepancy between *in vitro* phenotypes and *in vivo* tumorigenicity was found in cell lines established after transfer of viral DNA linked to a selectable drug-resistant gene (74). In the presence of the drug, resistant colonies scored with a frequency of 10- to 20-fold higher than that of dense foci in normal medium. On the basis of morphology and growth, lines established from resistant colonies were indistinguishable from original cells in that they maintained an extended, flat morphology and organized cytoskeletal structures. In 10% serum, they grew to a low saturation density, did not grow in agarose medium, and could not survive in the presence of 0.5% serum. In selective medium, cells maintained autonomous copies of the plasmid DNA, without any detectable rearrangement.

When passaged in cell culture, these lines exhibited an unusually high rate of spontaneous oncogenic transformation, as was determined by monitoring the appearance of dense foci in serial subcultures. Transformation occurred more frequently after exposure to a tumor promoter (TPA), which had no effect on the original FR3T3 cells. On injection into syngeneic rats, these apparently normal cells induced the formation of tumors, but only after latency periods of several months. These tumors were still more invasive than those induced by phenotypically transformed cells.

In addition to these *stage 1* cells, selected on the basis of their drug resistance, and *stage 2* transformants, obtained by direct selection for focus formation or by spontaneous transformation of stage 1 lines, two other phenotypes have been identified among cell lines established *in vitro* from the tumors produced by stage 1 and stage 2 cell lines (26) (Table 4). They were sufficiently reproducible to be considered *stages 3* and *4* of the tumoral evolution induced by BPV1 in fibroblasts.

Stage 3 corresponds to lines established earlier in culture from tumors developed from stage 2 cells. Compared with the latter, they had acquired two properties usually associated with tumorigenic potential: plating in agarose medium and secretion of plasminogen activator. It was striking, however, to observe that these tumor-derived cells still maintained a flat morphology, organized cytoskeletal structures, and needed high serum concentrations for growth in culture (52).

Stage 4 corresponds to cell lines selected directly from stage 1 by tumoral growth. They exhibited the same growth properties as stage 3 cell lines and even higher levels of tumorigenicity. In contrast to all other BPV1 transformants, they had undergone important morphological changes, with a complete disruption of cytoskeletal structures.

Southern blot analysis revealed the presence at stages 3 and 4 of autonomous copies of the viral DNA. Unlike observations at stages 1 and 2, however, these plasmidial molecules had often undergone rearrangements. These were of a limited extent at stage 3, a number of lines producing in fact the same profile as the original transformant. By contrast, the more advanced stage 4 cells always showed highly rearranged patterns and variable numbers of copies, some of them possibly integrated into the host genome. In one stage 4 line, no viral DNA could be evidenced. The changes characteristic of stage 4—loss of cytoskeletal structure and rearrangement of the viral DNA—were sometimes observed, although less pronounced, in cell lines derived from the short-latency tumors (stage 3).

Multistep transformation by BPV1 *in vitro* offers some interesting analogies to the malignant evolution of the tumors associated with human papillomaviruses. Association starts in both cases with nearly normal phenotypes from which different types of tumor cells will eventually emerge, depending on the selective pressure applied. On growth *in vivo,* stage 1 cells produced stage 4 progeny only after long latency periods, suggesting that, as in naturally occurring cancers, it implies the progressive accumulation of a number of rare events. Transit *in vitro* through stages 2 and 3 might allow a more detailed analysis of this evolution.

One of the most important questions that we may hope to answer by using experimental systems in parallel with further analysis of the natural history of papilloma-associated neoplasias is the relative role in this progression of viral and cellular oncogenic determinants. It is of course more than likely (although not yet rigorously demonstrated) that maintenance of transformation at the earliest stages depends on the expression of viral genes. Further transitions *in vitro* from stage 1 to stages 2 to 4 may be related to changes of either a quantitative or a qualitative nature in the expression of a series of viral oncogenes. Alternatively, cellular oncogenes may be activated that would either cooperate with the viral gene(s) or, at some point in the progression, completely substitute for the viral functions. Interest in relatively simple *in vitro* experimental systems is mainly due to the fact that present-day genetic technologies may allow us to perform critical experiments to answer such questions. Some of these experiments are presently under way in our laboratory and in others, but a few preliminary observations can be made. By contrast with the maintenance of unrearranged viral genomes in the early stages, extensive rearrangements, integration, and even loss of the viral DNA sequences have been observed in the terminal evolution of both human and animal cancers (12,66) or in cultures from cervical carcinomas (8), as well in BPV1 stage 4 trans-

TABLE 4. *BPV1-transformed FR3T3 derivatives*

			Phenotype in culture		
Stage	Select	From	Cell structure	Growth control	TPA reactivity
0	None	FR3T3	Flat	Normal	No
1	G418	FR3T3	Flat	Normal	Yes
2	Foci	FR3T3 or Stage 1	Flat	Focus formation Serum dependent Agar growth; − to ±	
3	Tumor	Stage 2	Flat	Agar growth; + + + Serum dependent	
4	Tumor	Stage 1	Compact		

formed cells. This might suggest that cellular determinants are important in the maintenance of advanced tumorigenic states (98). The other possibly relevant observation is that properties of BPV1 transformants are different in many important respects of the "tumor-associated transformation properties" previously described. Maintenance of organized cytoskeletal structures and serum dependence were not expected in cells endowed with a high tumorigenic potential, and that makes these transformants different from those established from the same cells after transformation with polyomaviruses or activated *ras* oncogenes. Assuming that cellular oncogenes are involved, we might be dealing with genes or a combination of genes different from those found in other tumor and transformed cells. It would then be of interest to compare the rat stage 3 and 4 lines and human carcinomas.

DISCUSSION

In the two families of oncogenic viruses considered in this review, viral genes responsible for cell transformation are involved in the establishment of the earliest detectable stages of tumoral progression ["subthreshold neoplastic states" (103)] in which a cell, still normal in many of its properties, will show the "ability to react to an extrinsic stimulus, called 'responsiveness' " (38). Responsiveness of *plt-* or *myc*-immortalized cells and of stage 1 BPV1 transformants was evidenced by their high rates of spontaneous transformation (in fact, reaction to unknown stimuli) and their response to TPA (18,25), and from a genetic point of view, by their susceptibility to a variety of cellular and viral oncogenes. This variety by itself [see Müller and Verma (79) for review] sufficiently indicates the multiplicity of routes through which a cell that starts from such a "high-risk state" can pro-

	Tumorigenicity	
Latency	Invasiveness	Metastasis
>8 Months		
3–5 Months	+	+
4–8 Weeks	+	+
8–10 Days	+	+ +
2–4 Days	+	+ +

ceed to malignancy. With respect to dependence on viral functions, two situations are expected and were in fact observed in the cases under review: either viral oncogenes continue to be active at one or several further stages (polyoma transformants) or they are at some point in the progression relayed by activated cellular oncogenes (some SV40-induced tumors). The choice between these two situations is a critical question in viral oncology. It cannot be answered yet for Papillomaviruses. One of the significant results expected from studies presently in progress in a number of laboratories is precisely that of the genetic determination of the shifts from early proliferative lesions to advanced malignant neoplasias.

Improving our knowledge of the very first step(s) of the transformation process is very important. Identifying the earliest manifestation of the disease, in most instances not accessible to the clinician, may open new diagnostic and, eventually, therapeutic strategies. This requires the extensive use of *in vitro* model systems, where we can follow the transition from a truly normal cell (therefore necessarily a cell in primary culture) to the immediate next step. One such early stage is observed in REF cells immortalized by the *plt, myc,* and E1A oncogenes, and its possible generality is still a matter of speculation. One view, overly optimistic, would be that all neoplastic diseases start with a stage comparable to immortalized rodent cells, with only some phenotypic variations, depending on the cell type and species. Available data suggest that this is not the case, because the properties conferred on the same rodent cells by *plt* or *myc* and by BPV1 differ in several important respects: The two most characteristic phenotypes associated with the former—continuous growth in culture and serum independence—were not observed after transfer of BPV1 DNA (25,52). How many more such early stages and transformation routes, how many distinct cases dependent on the specific properties of a differentiated cell type, and eventually, what all these early transformation stages may have in common remain to be determined.

ACKNOWLEDGMENTS

We are indebted to M. J. Gonzalez for help in the preparation of the manuscript.

REFERENCES

1. Androhy, E.J., Schiller, J.T., and Lowy, D.R. (1985): Identification of the protein encoded by the E6 transforming gene of bovine Papillomaviruses. *Science*, 230:442–445.

1a. Asselin, C., Gélinas, C., and Bastin, M. (1983): Role of the three polyoma virus early proteins in tumorigenesis. *Mol. Cell. Biol.*, 3:1451–1457.

2. Baird, P.J. (1983): Serological evidence of the association of papillomavirus and cervical neoplasia. *Lancet*, 2:17–18.

3. Benjamin, T.L. (1984): The polyoma hr-t gene: An "oncogene" with a purpose. In: *Cancer Cells, Vol. 2*, pp. 117–122. Cold Spring Harbor Laboratory, Cold Spring Harbor, New York.

4. Binétruy, B., Meneguzzi, G., Breathnach, R., and Cuzin, F. (1982): Recombinant DNA molecules comprising bovine papilloma virus type 1 DNA linked to plasmid DNA are maintained in a plasmidial state both in rodent fibroblasts and in bacterial cells. *EMBO J.*, 1:621–628.

5. Boiron, M., Levy, J.P., Thomas, M., Friedman, J.C., and Bernard, J. (1964): Some properties of bovine papilloma virus. *Nature*, 201:423–424.

6. Boiron, M., Thomas, M., and Chenialle, P.H. (1965): A biological property of deoxyribonucleic acid extracted from bovine papilloma virus. *Virology*, 52:150–153.

7. Bolen, J.B., Thiele, C.J., Israel, M.A., Yonemoto, W., Lipsich, L.A., and Brugge, J.S. (1984): Enhancement of cellular *src* gene product associated tyrosyl kinase activity following polyoma virus infection and transformation. *Cell*, 38:767–777.

8. Boshart, M., Gissmann, L., Ikenberg, H., Kleinheinz, A., Scheurlen, W., and zur Hausen, H. (1984): A new type of papillomavirus DNA, its presence in genital cancer biopsies and in cell lines derived from cervical cancer. *EMBO J.*, 3:1151–1157.

9. Brady, J., Bolen, J.B., Radonovich, M., Salzman, N., and Khoury, G. (1984): Stimulation of simian virus 40 late gene expression by simian virus 40 tumor antigen. *Proc. Natl. Acad. Sci. U.S.A.*, 81:2040–2044.

10. Breitburd, F., Favre, M., Zoorob, R., Fortin, D., and Orth, G. (1981): Detection and characterization of viral genomes and search for tumoral antigens in two hamster cell lines derived from tumors induced by bovine papillomavirus. *Int. J. Cancer*, 27:693–702.

11. Buchman, A.R., Burnett, L., and Berg, P. (1980): The SV40 nucleotide sequence. In: *Molecular Biology of Tumor Viruses. II*, J. Tooze, ed., 2nd. ed., pp. 799–829. Cold Spring Harbor Laboratory, Cold Spring Harbor, New York.

12. Campo, M.S., Moar, M.H., Sartirana, M.L., Kennedy, I.M., and Jarrett, W.F.H. (1985): The presence of bovine papillomavirus type 4 DNA is not required for the progression to, or the maintenance of, the malignant state in cancers of the alimentary canal in cattle. *EMBO J.*, 4:1819–1825.

12a. Cerni, C., Mougneau, E., Zerlin, M., Julius, M., Marcu, K.B., and Cuzin, F. (1986): C-*myc* and functionally related oncogenes induce both high rates of sister chromatid exchange and abnormal karotypes in rat fibroblasts. *Curr. Top. Microbiol. Immunol. (in press)*.

13. Chen, E.Y., Howley, P.M., Levinson, A.D., and Seeburg, P.H. (1982): The primary structure and genetic organization of the bovine papillomavirus type 1 genome. *Nature*, 299:529–534.

14. Clertant, P., and Cuzin, F. (1982): Covalent affinity labeling by periodate-oxidized (-^{32}P)ATP of the large-T proteins of polyoma and SV40 viruses. *J. Biol. Chem.*, 257:6300–6305.

15. Clertant, P., Gaudray, P., May, E., and Cuzin, F. (1984): The nucleotide binding site detected by affinity labeling in the large T proteins of polyoma and SV40 viruses is distinct from their ATPase catalytic site. *J. Biol. Chem.*, 259:15196–15203.

16. Clertant, P., and Seif, I. (1984): A common function for polyoma virus large-T and papillomavirus E1 proteins? *Nature*, 311:276–279.

17. Cogen, B. (1978): Virus-specific early RNA in 3T6 cells infected by a tsA mutant of polyoma virus. *Virology*, 85:222–230.

18. Connan, G., Rassoulzadegan, M., and Cuzin, F. (1985): Focus formation in rat fibroblasts exposed to a tumor promoter after transfer of polyoma *plt* and *myc* oncogenes. *Nature,* 314:277–279.
19. Coulier, F., Imbert, J., Albert, J., Jeunet, E., Lawrence, J.J., Crawford, L., and Birg, F. (1985): Permanent expression of p53 in FR 3T3 rat cells but cell cycle-dependent association with large T antigen in simian virus 40 transformants. *EMBO J.,* 4:3413–3418.
20. Courtneidge, S.A. (1985): Activation of the pp60^{c-src} kinase by middle-T antigen binding or by dephosphorylation. *EMBO J.,* 4:1471–1478.
21. Courtneidge, S.A., and Smith, A.E. (1983): Polyoma virus transforming protein associates with the product of the *c-src* cellular gene. *Nature,* 303:435–439.
22. Crawford, l. (1982): The origins of p53 in relation to transformation. In: *Advances in Viral Oncology,* edited by G. Klein, Vol. 2, pp. 3–21. Raven Press, New York.
23. Crum, C.P., Mitao, M., Levine, R.U., and Silverstein, S. (1985): Cervical papillomaviruses segregate within morphologically distinct precancerous lesions. *J. Virol.,* 54:675–681.
24. Cuzin, F. (1984): The polyoma virus oncogenes: Coordinated functions of three distinct proteins in the transformation of rodent cells in culture. *Biochem. Biophys. Acta,* 781:193–204.
25. Cuzin, F., Meneguzzi, G., Binétruy, B., Cerni, C., Connan, G., Grisoni, M., and de Lapeyrière, O. (1985): Stepwise tumoral progression in rodent fibroblasts transformed with bovine papilloma virus type 1 (BPV1) DNA. In: *Papilloma viruses: Molecular and Clinical Aspects, Vol. 32* (U.C.L.A. Symposia, Molecular and Cellular Biology), edited by P.M. Howley and T.R. Broker, pp. 473–486. A.R. Liss, New York.
26. Cuzin, F., Rassoulzadegan, M., and Lemieux, L. (1984): Multigenic control of tumorigenesis: Three distinct oncogenes are required for transformation of rat embryo fibroblasts by polyoma virus. *Cancer Cells, Cold Spring Harbor,* 2:109–116.
27. Danos, O., Katinka, M., and Yaniv, M. (1982): Human papillomavirus la complete DNA sequence: A novel type of genome organization among Papovaridae. *EMBO J.,* 1:231–236.
28. Danos, O., and Yaniv, M. (1983): Structure and function of papillomavirus genomes. In: *Advances in Viral Oncology,* edited by G. Klein, Vol. 3, pp. 59–81. Raven Press, New York.
29. de Lapeyrière, O., Hayot, B., Imbert, J., Courcoul, M., Arnaud, M., and Birg, F. (1984): Cell lines derived from tumors induced in syngeneic rats by FR 3T3 SV40 transformants no longer synthesize the early viral proteins. *Virology,* 135:74–86.
30. Delmas, V., Bastien, C., Scherneck, S., and Feunteun, J. (1985): A new member of the polyomavirus family: The hamster papovavirus. Complete nucleotide sequence and transformation properties. *EMBO J.,* 4:1279–1286.
31. Deppert, W., and Henning, R. (1979): SV40 T-antigen-related molecules on the surface of adenovirus-2-SV40 hybrid-virus-infected HeLa cells and on SV40-transformed cells. *Cold Spring Harbor Symp. Quant. Biol.,* 44:225–234.
32. Dilworth, S.M., Cowie, A., Kamen, R.I., and Griffin, B.E. (1984): DNA binding activity of polyoma virus large-tumor antigen *Proc. Natl. Acad. Sci. U.S.A.,* 81:1941–1945.
33. DiMaio, D., Metherall, J., Neary, K., and Guralski, D. (1985): Genetic analysis of cell transformation by bovine papillomavirus. In: *Papillomaviruses: Molecular and Clinical Aspects, Vol. 32 (U.C.L.A. Symposia, Molecular and Cellular Biology),* edited by P.M. Howley and T.R. Broker, pp. 431–456. A.R. Liss, New York.
34. Dunn, A.E., and Ogilvie, M.M. (1968): Intranuclear virus particles in human genital wart tissue: Observation on the ultrastructure of epidermal layer. *J. Ultrastruct. Res.,* 22:282–295.
35. Dürst, M., Gissmann, L., Ikenberg, H., and zur Hansen, H. (1983): A papillomavirus DNA from a cervical carcinoma and its prevalence in cancer biopsies from different geographic regions. *Proc. Natl. Acad. Sci. U.S.A.,* 60:3812–3815.
36. Elihyahu, D., Raz, A., Gruss, P., Givol, D., and Oren, M. (1984): Participation of p53 cellular tumor antigen in transformation of normal embryonic cells. *Nature,* 312:646–649.
37. Fenton, R.G., and Basilico, C. (1982): Changes in the topography of early region transcription during polyoma virus lytic infection. *Proc. Natl. Acad. Sci. U.S.A.,* 79:7142–7146.
38. Foulds, L. (1954): The experimental study of tumor progression: A review. *Cancer Res.,* 14:327–339.
39. Francke, B., and Eckhart, W. (1973): Polyoma gene function required for viral DNA synthesis. *Virology,* 55:127–135.
40. Friedman, T., Esty, A., La Porte, P., and Deininger, P. (1979): The nucleotide sequence and genome organization of the polyoma virus early region: Extensive nucleotide and aminoacid homology with SV40. *Cell,* 17:715–724.

41. Gaudray, P., Clertant, P., and Cuzin, F. (1980): ATP phosphohydrolase (ATPase) activity of a polyoma virus T antigen. *Eur. J. Biochem.*, 109:553–560.
42. Gaudray, P., Tyndall, C., Kamen, R., and Cuzin, F. (1981): The high-affinity binding site on polyoma virus DNA for the viral large-T protein. *Nucl. Acid Res.*, 9:5697–5710.
43. Giri, I., Danos, O., and Yaniv, M. (1985): Genomic structure of the cottontail rabbit (Shope) papillomavirus. *Proc. Natl. Acad. Sci. U.S.A.*, 82:1580–1584.
44. Gissmann, L. (1985): Papillomaviruses and their association with cancer in animals and in man. *Cancer Surveys*, 3:160–181.
45. Gissmann, L., Diehl, V., Schultz-Coulon, H.J., and zur Hausen, H. (1982): Molecular cloning and characterization of human papillomavirus DNA derived from a laryngeal papilloma. *J. Virol.*, 44:393–400.
46. Gissmann, L., and Schwartz, E. (1985): Cloning of papillomavirus DNA. In: *Developments in Molecular Virology, Vol. 5. Recombinant DNA Research and Virus*, edited by Y. Becker, pp. 173–197. Martinus Nijhoff Publ. Hingham, Massachusetts.
47. Gissmann, L., Wolnik, L., Ikenberg, H., Koldovsky, U., Schnurch, H.G., and zur Hausen, H. (1983): Human papillomavirus types 6 and 11 DNA sequences in genital and laryngeal papillomas and in some cervical cancers. *Proc. Natl. Acad. Sci. U.S.A.*, 80:560–563.
48. Graf, T., and Stéhelin, D. (1982): Avian leukemia viruses: Oncogenes and genome structure. *Biochem. Biophys. Acta*, 651:245–271.
49. Green, M., Brachmann, K.H., Sanders, P.R., Lowenstein, P.M., Freel, J.H., Eisinger, M., and Switlyk, S.A. (1982): Isolation of a human papillomavirus from a patient with epidermodysplasia verruciformis: Presence of related viral DNA genomes in human urogenital tumors. *Proc. Natl. Acad. Sci. U.S.A.*, 79.4437–4441.
50. Griffin, B.E., and Karran, L. (1984): Immortalization of monkey epithelial cells by specific fragments of Epstein-Barr virus DNA. *Nature*, 309:78–82.
51. Griffin, B.E., Soeda, E., Barrell, B.G., and Staden, R. (1980): Sequence and analysis of polyoma virus DNA. In: *Molecular Biology of Tumor Viruses. II*, edited by J. Tooze, 2nd ed., pp. 831–895. Cold Spring Harbor Laboratory, Cold Spring Harbor, New York.
52. Grisoni, M., Meneguzzi, G., de Lapeyrière, O., Binétruy, B., Rassoulzadegan, M., and Cuzin, F. (1984): The transformed phenotype in culture and tumorigenecity of Fischer rat fibroblast cells (FR3T3) transformed with Bovine papilloma virus type 1. *Virology*, 135:406–416.
53. Hand, R. (1981): Functions of T antigens of SV40 and polyoma virus. *Biochem. Biophys. Acta*, 651:1–24.
54. Ikenberg, H., Gissmann, L., Gross, G., Grussendorf-Conèn, E.I., and zur Hausen, H. (1983): Human papillomavirus type 16-related DNA in genital Bowen's disease and in Bowenoid papulosis. *Int. J. Cancer*, 32:563–565.
55. Ito, Y. (1980): Organization and expression of the genome of polyoma virus. in: *Advances in Viral Oncology*, edited by G. Klein, pp. 447–480. Raven Press, New York.
56. Ito, Y., Spurr, N., and Dulbecco, R. (1977): Characterization of polyoma virus T antigen. *Proc. Natl. Acad. Sci. U.S.A.*, 74:1259–1263.
57. Jariwalla, R.J., Aurelian, L., and Ts'o, P.O. (1984): Immortalization and neoplastic transformation of normal diploid cells by defined cloned fragments of herpes simplex virus type 2. *Proc. Natl. Acad. Sci. U.S.A.*, 80:5902–5906.
58. Jarrett, W.F.H., McNeil, P.E., Grimshaw, W.T.R., Selman, I.E., and McIntryre, W.I.M. (1978): High-incidence area of cattle cancer with a possible interaction between an environmental carcinogen and a papilloma virus. *Nature*, 274:215–217.
59. Kremsdorf, D., Jablonska, S., Favre, M., and Orth, G. (1983): Human papilloma viruses associated with epidermodysplasia verruciformis. *J. Virol.*, 48:340–351.
60. Kress, M., May, E., Cassingena, R., and May, P.(1979): Simian virus 40-transformed cells express new species of proteins precipitable by anti-simian virus 40 tumor serum. *J. Virol.*, 31:472–483.
61. Lancaster, W., and Olson, C. (1982): Animal papilloma viruses. *Microbiolog. Rev.*, 46:191–207.
62. Land, H., Parada, L.F., and Weinberg, R.A. (1983): Tumorigenic conversion of primary embryo fibroblasts requires at least two cooperating oncogenes. *Nature*, 304:596–602.
63. Lane, D.P., and Crawford, L.V. (1979): T antigen is bound to a host protein in SV40-transformed cells. *Nature*, 278:261–263.
64. Lanford, R.E., and Butel, J. (1979): Antigenic relationship of SV40 early proteins to purified large-T polypeptide. *Virology*, 97:295–306.

65. La Porta, R.F., and Taichman, L.B. (1982): Human papilloma viral DNA replicates as a stable episome in cultured epidermal keratinocytes. *Proc. Natl. Acad. Sci, U.S.A.*, 79:3393–3397.
66. Lehn, H., Krieg, P., and Sauer, G. (1985): Papilloma virus genomes in human cervical tumors: analysis of their transcriptional activity. *Proc. Natl. Acad. Sci. U.S.A.*, 82:5540–5544.
67. Levine, A.J., Oren, M., Reich, N., and Sarnow, P. (1982): The mechanisms regulating the levels of the cellular p53 tumor antigen in transformed cells. in: *Advances in Viral Oncology,* edited by G. Klein, Vol. 2, pp. 81–102. Raven Press, New York.
68. Linzer, D.I.H., and Levine, A.J. (1979): Characterization of a 54K-dalton cellular SV40 tumor antigen present in SV40-transformed cells and uninfected embryonal carcinoma cells. *Cell,* 22:917–927.
69. Lusky, M., and Botchan, M.R. (1984): Characterization of the bovine papilloma virus plasmid maintenance sequences. *Cell,* 36:391–401.
70. McCance, D.J., Walker, P.G., Dyson, J.L., Coleman, D.V., and Singer, A. (1983): Presence of human papillomavirus DNA sequences in cervical intraepithelial neoplasia. *Br. Med. J.,* 287:784–788.
71. McVay, P., Fretz, M., Wettstein, F., Stevens, J., and Ito, Y. (1982): Integrated Shope virus DNA is present and transcribed in the transplantable rabbit tumour V_x-7. *Gen. Virol.,* 60:271–278.
72. Meisels, A., and Fortin, R. (1976):Condylomatous lesions of the cervix and vagina. I. Cytologic patterns. *Acta Cytol.,* 20:505–509.
73. Meisels, A., and Morin, C. (1981): Human papillomavirus and cancer of the uterine cervix. *Gynecol. Oncol.,* 12:111–123.
74. Meneguzzi, G., Binétruy, B., Grisoni, M., and Cuzin, F. (1984): Plasmidial maintenance in rodent fibroblasts of a BPV1-pBR322 shuttle vector without immediately apparent oncogenic transformation of the recipient cells. *EMBO J.,* 3:365–371.
75. Mercer, W.E., Nelson, D., DeLeo, A.B., Old, L.J., and Baserga, R. (1982): Microinjection of monoclonal antibody to protein p53 inhibits serum-induced DNA synthesis in 3T3 cells. *Proc. Natl. Acad. Sci. U.S.A.,* 79:6309–6312.
76. Milner, J., and Milner, S. (1981): A possible role for 53 K in normal cells. *Virology,* 112:785–788.
77. Mougneau, E., Lemieux, L., Rassoulzadegan, M., and Cuzin, F. (1984): Biological activities of the v-*myc* and of rearranged c-*myc* oncogenes in rat fibroblast cells in culture. *Proc. Natl. Acad. Sci. U.S.A.,* 81:5758–5762.
78. Mounts, P, Shah, K.V., and Kashima, H. (1982): Viral etiology of juvenile- and adult-onset squamous papilloma of the larynx. *Proc. Natl. Acad. Sci. U.S.A.,* 79:5425–5429.
79. Müller, R., and Verma, I.M. (1984): Expression of cellular oncogenes. *Curr. Top. Microbiol. Immunol.,* 112:73–115.
80. Nakabayashi, Y., Chattopadhyay, S.K., and Lowy, D.R. (1983): The transforming function of bovine papillomavirus DNA. *Proc. Natl. Acad. Sci. U.S.A.,* 80:5832–5836.
81. Nilsson, S.V., and Magnusson, G. (1984): Activities of polyomavirus large-T-antigen proteins expressed by mutant genes. *J. Virol.,* 51:768–775.
82. Oriel, J.D., and Almeida, J.D. (1970): Demonstration of virus particles in human genital warts. *Br. J. Vener. Dis.,* 46:37–42.
83. Orth, G. (1986): Epidermodysplasia verruciformis: A model for understanding the oncogenicity of human papillomviruses. In: *Papillomaviruses, Vol. 120,* edited by P. London, pp. 157–169. Wiley, New York.
84. Orth, G., Breitburd, F., and Favre, M. (1978): Evidence for antigenic determinants shared by the structural polypeptides of (Shope) rabbit papillomavirus and human papillomavirus type 1. *Virology,* 91:243–255.
85. Orth, G., and Favre, M. (1985): Human papillomaviruses, biochemical and biologic properties. *Clin. Derm.,* 3(4):27–42.
86. Orth, G., Favre, M., Bretburd, F., Croissant, O., Jablonska, S., Obalek, S., Jarzabek-Chorzelska, M., and Rzesa, G. (1980): Epidermodysplasia verruciformis: A model for the role of papillomaviruses in human cancer. *Cold Spring harbor Conf. cell Proliferation,* 7:259–282.
87. Orth, G., Jablonska, S., Jarzabek-Chorzelska, M., Obalek, S., Rzesa, G., Fabre, M., and Croissant, O. (1979): Characteristics of the lesions and risk of malignant conversion associated with the type of human papilloma virus involved in epidermodysplasia verruciformis. *Cancer Res.,* 39:1074–1082.

88. Ostrow, R.S., Bender, M., Nimura, M., Seki, T., Kawashima, M., Pass, F., and Faras, A.J. (1982): Human papillomavirus DNA in cutaneous primary and metastasized squamous cell carcinomas from patients with epidermodysplasia verruciformis. *Proc. Natl. Acad. Sci. U.S.A.,* 79:1634–1638.

89. Parada, L.F., Land, H., Weinberg, R.A., Wolf, D., and Rotter, V. (1984): Cooperation between gene-encoding p53 tumor antigen and *ras* in cellular transformation. *Nature,* 312:649–651.

90. Parker, R.C., Varmus, H.E., and Bishop, J.M. (1984): Expression of v-*src* and chicken c-*src* in rat cells demonstrates qualitative differences between pp60^{v-src} and pp60^{c-src}. *Cell,* 37:131–139.

91. Pfister, H. (1984): Biology and biochemistry of papilloma viruses. *Rev. Physiol. Biochem. Pharmacol.,* 99:111–181.

92. Purola, E., and Savia, E. (1977): Cytology of gynecologic condyloma acuminatum. *Acta Cytol.,* 21:26–31.

93. Rassoulzadegan, M., Cowie, A., Carr, A., Glaichenhaus, N., Kamen, R., and Cuzin, F. (1982): The roles of individual polyoma virus early proteins in oncogenic transformation. *Nature,* 300:713–718.

94. Rassoulzadegan, M., Mougneau, E., Perbal, B., Gaudray, P., Birg, F., and Cuzin, F. (1980): Host–virus interactions critical for cellular transformation by polyoma virus and simian virus 40. *Cold Spring Harbor Symp. Quant. Biol.,* 44:333–342.

95. Rassoulzadegan, M., Naghashfar, Z., Cowie, A., Carr, A., Grisoni, M., Kamen, R., and Cuzin, F. (1983): Expression of the large T protein of polyoma virus promotes the establishment in culture of "normal" rodent fibroblast cells. *Proc. Natl. Acad. Sci. U.S.A.,* 80:4354–4358.

96. Reich, N.C., and Levine, A.J. (1984): Growth regulation of a cellular tumor antigen, p53, in nontransformed cells. *Nature,* 308:199–201.

97. Reid, R., Laverty, C.R., Coppleson, M., Isarangkul, W., and Hills, E. (1980): Noncondylomatous cervical wart virus infection. *Obstet. Gynecol.,* 55:476–483.

98. Riou, G., Barrois, M., Dutronquay, V., and Orth, G. (1985): Papilloma viruses: Molecular and clinical aspects. In: *Papillomaviruses: Molecular and Clinical Aspects, Vol. 32.,* edited by P.M. Howley and T.R. Broker, pp. 47–56. *Symposia Molecular and Cellular Biology,* A.R. Liss, New York.

99. Risser, R., and Pollack, R. (1974): A nonselective analysis of SV40 transformation of mouse 3T3 cells. *Virology,* 59:477–489.

100. Rous, P., and Beard, J.W. (1934): A virus-induced mammalian growth with the characters of a tumor (the Shope) rabbit papilloma. *J. Exp. Med.,* 60:701–722.

101. Rous, P., and Beard, J.W. (1935): The progression to carcinomas of virus-induced papillomas (Shope). *J. Exp. Med.,* 62:523–548.

102. Rous, R., and Friedwald, W.F. (1944): The effect of chemical carcinogens on virus-induced rabbit carcinomas. *J. Exp. Med.,* 79:511–537.

103. Rous, P., and Kidd, J.G. (1941): Conditional neoplasms and subthreshold neoplastic states. *J. Exp. Med.,* 73:365–389.

104. Ruley, H.E. (1983): Adenovirus early-region 1A enables viral and cellular transforming genes to transform primary cells in culture. *Nature,* 304:602–606.

105. Ruley, H.E., Moomaw, J.F., and Maruyama, K. (1984): Avian myelocytomatosis virus *myc* and adenovirus early-region E1A promote the *in vitro* establishment of cultured primary cells. *Cancer Cells, Cold Spring Harbor,* 2:481–486.

106. Rundell, K. (1982): Presence in growth-arrested cells of cellular proteins that interact with simian virus 40 small-t antigen. *J. Virol.,* 42:1135–1137.

107. Rundell, K., Major, E.O., and Lampert, M. (1981): Association of cellular 56,000- and 32,000-molecular-weight proteins with BK virus and polyoma virus t-antigens. *J. Virol.,* 37:1090–1093.

108. Schiller, J.T., Vass, W.C., and Lowy, D.R. (1984): Identification of a second transforming region in bovine papilloma virus DNA. *Proc. Natl. Acad. Sci. U.S.A.,* 81:7880–7884.

109. Schwarz, E., Durst, M., Demankowski, C., Lattermann, O., Zech, R., Wolfsperger, R., Shuai, S., and zur Hausen, H. (1983): DNA sequence genome organization of genital human papillomavirus type 6b. *EMBO J.,* 2:2341–2348.

110. Schwarz, E., Freese, U.K., Gissmann, L., Mayer, W., Roggenbuck, B., Stremlau, A., and zur Hausen, H. (1985): Structure and transcription of human papillomavirus sequences in cervical carcinoma cells. *Nature,* 314:111–114.

111. Seedorf, K., Krämmer, G., Dürst, M., Suhai, S., and Röwekamp, W.G. (1985): Human papillomavirus type 16 DNA sequence. *Virology,* 145:181–185.

112. Seif, R., Seif, I., and Wantyghem, J. (1983): Rat cells transformed by simian virus 40 give rise to tumor cells which contain no viral proteins and often no viral DNA. *Mol. Cell. Biol.*, 3:1138–1145.

113. Sharma, S., Rodgers, L., Brandsma, J., Gething, M.J., and Sambrook, J. (1985): SV40 T antigen and the exocytic pathway. *EMBO J.*, 4:1479–1490.

114. Smith, K.T., and Campo, M.S. (1985): The biology of papillomaviruses and their role in oncogenesis. *Anticancer Res.*, 5:31–48.

115. Soeda, E., Arrand, J.R., Smolar, N., Walsh, J.E., and Griffin, B.E. (1980): Coding potential and regulatory signals of the polyoma virus genome. *Nature*, 283:445–453.

115a. Spandidos, D.A., and Wilkie, N.M. (1984): Malignant transformation of early passage rodent cells by a single mutated human oncogene. *Nature*, 310:469–475.

116. Spradbrow, P.B., and Hoffmann, D. (1980): Bovine ocular squamous cell carcinoma. *Vet. Bull.*, 50:449–459.

117. Spriggs, A.I. (1981): Natural history of cervical dysplasia. *Clin. Obstet. Gynecol.*, 8:65–79.

118. Stewart, S.E. (1960): The polyoma virus. *Adv. Virus Res.*, 7:61–90.

119. Todaro, G.J., and Green, H. (1963): Quantitative studies on the growth of mouse embryo cells in culture and their development into established lines. *J. Cell Biol.*, 17:299–313.

120. Treisman, R., Novak, U., Favaloro, J., and Kamen, R. (1981): Transformation of rat cells by an altered polyoma virus genome expressing only the middle-T protein. *Nature*, 292:595–600.

121. Van den Elsen, P., de Pater, S., Houweling, A., van der Veer, J., and van der Eb, A. (1982): The relationship between region E1a and E1b of human adenoviruses in cell transformation. *Gene*, 18:175–185.

122. Vanselow, B.A., and Spradbrow, P.B. (1982): Papillomaviruses, papillomas, and squamous cell carcinomas in sheep. *Vet. Rec.*, 110:561–562.

123. Vogt, M., and Dulbecco, R. (1963): Steps in the neoplastic transformation of hamster embryo cells by polyoma virus. *Proc. Natl. Acad. Sci. U.S.A.*, 49:171–179.

124. Vogt, M., and Dulbecco, R. (1963): Properties of cells transformed by polyoma virus. *Cold Spring Harbor Symp. Quant. Biol.*, 28:367–374.

125. Waldeck, W., Rösl, F., and Zentgraf, H. (1984): Origin of replication in episomal bovine papillomavirus type 1 DNA isolated from transformed cells. *EMBO J.*, 3:2173–2178.

126. Wettstein, F.O., and Stevens, J.G. (1982): Variable-sized free episomes of Shope papillomavirus DNA are present in all nonvirus-producing neoplasms, and integrated episomes are detected in some. *Proc. Natl. Acad. Sci. U.S.A.*, 79:790–794.

127. Yang, Y., Hearing, P., and Rundell, K. (1979): Cellular proteins associated with simian virus 40 early-gene products in newly infected cells. *J. Virol.*, 32:147–154.

128. Yang, Y.-C., Okayama, H., and Howley, P.M. (1985): Bovine papillomavirus contains multiple transforming genes. *Proc. Natl. Acad. Sci. U.S.A.*, 82:1030–1034.

129. Zachaw, K.R., Ostrow, R.S., Bender, M., Watts, S., Okagaki, T., Pass, F., and Faras, A.J. (1982): Detection of human papillomavirus DNA in anogenital neoplasias. *Nature*, 300:771–773.

130. zur Hausen, H. (1977): Human papilloma viruses and their possible role in squamous cell carcinomas. *Curr. Top. Microbiol. Immunol.*, 78:1–30.

Advances in Viral Oncology, Volume 6, edited by
George Klein. Raven Press, New York © 1987.

Multiple Cell-Derived Sequences in Single Retroviral Genomes

Klaus Bister

*Otto-Warburg-Laboratorium, Max-Planck-Institut für Molekulare Genetik,
D-1000 Berlin 33 (Dahlem), Federal Republic of Germany*

Nondefective weakly oncogenic retroviruses carry on their genomes three genes essential for virus replication: *gag,* encoding the virion core proteins; *pol,* directing synthesis of the RNA-dependent DNA polymerase (reverse transcriptase); and *env,* specifying virion envelope glycoproteins. Highly oncogenic retroviruses contain transformation-specific sequences inserted into their genomes, in all but one case (Rous sarcoma virus) at the expense of replication-specific genes. The search for the origin of transformation-specific sequences in retroviral genomes led to the startling discovery of conserved cellular genes, which are closely related in their nucleotide sequence to retroviral transforming genes (or oncogenes) yet fulfill presumably essential physiological functions in the normal cell. Based on structural evidence, it appears almost certain that highly oncogenic retroviruses arose by recombination between replication-competent weakly oncogenic retroviruses and the apparent cellular progenitors of retroviral oncogenes. Hence, retroviral oncogenes, termed v-*onc* genes, represent transduced mutant alleles of cellular oncogenes, termed c-*onc* genes. The normal nononcogenic alleles of cellular oncogenes are also designated as protooncogenes, and the oncogenic mutant alleles as active oncogenes. Since protooncogenes are expressed in normal cells and hence are active genes, the term "active" oncogene refers to activation of oncogenic function. The transition from a normal allele to a transduced mutant allele with oncogenic function is always accompanied by multiple changes in gene structure and control of gene expression (13,118).

From classical and molecular oncology has emerged the idea that cancer is probably the final product of a multistep process, presumably involving multiple genes (30,61,67,112; see also *this volume*). Highly oncogenic retroviruses, which are apparently capable of transforming cells in a single step, may yet be compatible in their action with the concept of the multistep nature of carcinogenesis. It has been argued that the multiple changes in the evolution of retroviral oncogenes from their cellular progenitors may be analogous to the multiple stages in nonviral carcinogenesis (112). This may be particularly true in those cases where the genome of a highly oncogenic retrovirus apparently arose by recombination of a retroviral vector with more than one cellular component. The Kirsten and Harvey strains of murine sarcoma virus, for example, apparently arose by recombination between murine leukemia virus, the rat Kirsten or Harvey c-*ras* locus, respectively, and rat "30S" sequences. Although only the v-*ras* alleles are expressed as protein products and represent the transforming principle of these viruses,the 30S sequences may have played an essential role in the genesis of these interspecies recombinants (28). Other retroviruses contain in their genomes two cell-derived inserts that are both expressed as protein products, either independently or as a hybrid polyprotein. In these cases, both cell-derived components could be directly involved in the transforming activity of those viruses. Such viruses may represent the products of a natural selection for enhanced oncogenicity caused by additive, complementary, mutually modulating, or directly cooperative functions of two cell-derived inserts whose simultaneous and augmented expression is guaranteed by their presence on a single retroviral genome. However, in most cases of cotransduction of cellular sequences, only one of them is genetically well defined or derived from a cellular oncogene that has independently been transduced as a single oncogenic determinant in other retroviral isolates. Hence, the functional significance of the second cell-derived component, particularly if it encodes only minor domains of hybrid proteins, is difficult to assess, and cotransduction of cellular sequences in the genome of a highly oncogenic retrovirus does not necessarily imply that they all are authentic oncogenes capable of transforming normal cells as autonomous oncogenic determinants. In this chapter, I shall review structural and functional aspects of retroviral genomes carrying multiple cell-derived sequences that are expressed as protein products. Comprehensive reviews on the biochemistry and the molecular genetics of oncogenes may be found in Bister and Jansen (13) and Vamus (118).

COTRANSDUCED SEQUENCES ENCODING
SEPARATE PROTEIN PRODUCTS

There are two retroviral isolates that carry in their genomes cotransduced sequences encoding separate protein products. Both are species of the avian acute leukemia virus group: Avian erythroblastosis virus (AEV) strain R (or ES4) is a member of the AEV subgroup (defined by shared v-*erb*-B oncogenes) of acute leukemia viruses; and avian carcinoma virus MH2 belongs to the MC29 subgroup (defined by shared v-*myc* oncogenes) of acute leukemia viruses (9,11–13). Of particular interest is the genetic structure of the highly oncogenic virus MH2. MH2 is the only known retrovirus that contains in its genome two contransduced sequences, both of which have also been found in the form of autonomously oncogenic mutant alleles in independent retroviral isolates.

myc and *mil* in **MH2**

The genetic structure of MH2 (18,53,55,58) is depicted in Fig. 1. The MH2 genome contains a 5′ segment of the *gag* gene but no *pol* or *env* sequences. The v-*myc* allele of MH2 is located near the 3′ end of the genome, and it is separated from the partial *gag* gene by v-*mil,* the second oncogene of MH2. There are no viral sequences interspersed between the two cell-derived inserts. The MH2 v-*myc* allele contains a 5′ segment derived from intron sequences directly adjacent to the second c-*myc* exon, including the splice acceptor signal, and a short untranslated sequence of 39 nucleotides 3′ of the conserved translational termination codon (59,108,109). Hence, the entire coding domain of the c-*myc* gene contained within the second and third exons has been transduced into the MH2 genome. The nucleotide sequence of MH2 v-*myc* differs from that of chicken c-*myc* within the shared coding domain by single-nucleotide substitutions, leading to 27 amino acid exchanges in the predicted protein sequence, and by the deletion of four consecutive codons (Table 1). The expression of the MH2 v-*myc* allele is mediated by translation of a subgenomic mRNA species (Fig. 1), which is found in MH2-transformed cells in addition to genome-sized mRNA (86). The splicing process apparently utilizes the standard splice donor site located within the very 5′ coding domain of the *gag* gene of retroviruses from the avian leukosis sarcoma group (101) and the c-*myc*-derived splice acceptor site within the MH2 v-*myc* insert. Direct evidence

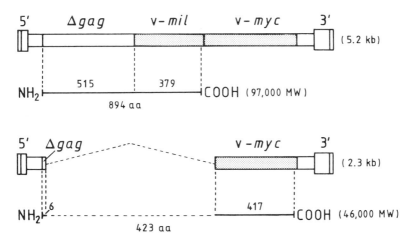

FIG. 1. Genetic structure of avian carcinoma virus MH2. Genome-sized and subgenomic mRNAs and their protein products are shown. On the RNA molecules, *open boxes* represent viral sequences, and *stippled boxes* represent transduced cell-derived sequences. The boxes marked 5′ and 3′ represent the RU5 and U3R terminal sequences, respectively, of viral RNA. Partial complements of virion genes are marked by Δ. The complexities of RNAs are given in kilobases (kb), and the sizes of proteins are shown in total numbers of amino acid residues (aa) and in calculated molecular weight (MW, in rounded numbers). The numbers of amino acid residues encoded by specific regions of translational units are also indicated.

TABLE 1. *Differences between chicken c-myc and retroviral v-myc alleles in nucleotide sequence and predicted amino acid sequence[a]*

Codon[b]	c-myc	v-myc (MC29)	v-myc (CMII)	v-myc (OK10)	v-myc (MH2)
005	GCC:Ala				GTC:Val
034	CTG:Leu				TCG:Ser[e]
040	GGC:Gly				AGC:Ser
046	CCC:Pro				CCA
061	ACG:Thr	ATG:Met		GCG:Ala	GCG:Ala
068	CGC:Arg				TGC:Cys
071	AGC:Ser				AAC:Asn
101	TTC:Phe				TCC:Ser
117	CAG:Gln				CGG:Arg
142	CAA:Gln				AAA:Lys
146	CGG:Arg	CAG:Gln[c]			
187	GAC:Asp				GGC:Gly
190	GAC:Asp				GGC:Gly
191	CCC:Pro				TCC:Ser
197	TAC:Tyr				TGC:Cys
200	AGC:Ser				GGC:Gly
201	GAG:Glu				AGG:Arg
203	GCC:Ala				GGC:Gly
204	CCG:Pro				- - -:—
205	CGG:Arg				- - -:—
206	GCC:Ala				- - -:—
207	GCC:Ala				- - -:—
212	AAC:Asn				GGC:Gly
221	ACG:Thr				GCG:Ala
225	ACC:Thr				GTC:Val[f]
226	AGC:Ser				GGC:Gly
227	AGC:Ser				GGC:Gly
228	GAC:Asp				GGC:Gly
230	GAA:Glu				GAG
257	AGC:Ser				GGC:Gly[g]
275	AAG:Lys				GAG:Glu
313	ATC:Ile				GTC:Val
325	TCA:Ser	TTA:Leu			
329	GAG:Glu				GTG:Val
335	ACG:Thr			ATG:Met	
350	AGT:Ser	CGT:Arg			
355	CGT:Arg				CGG
375	AAA:Lys				AGA:Arg
383	ATC:Ile	CTC:Leu			
389	AGA:Arg	AAA:Lys[d]			
390	CTA:Leu	CTG			CTG
407	AAA:Lys	AAC:Asn			
416	GCA:Ala		GAA:Glu		

[a]Based on sequence analyses from the following references: chicken c-*myc* (123); MC29 v-*myc* (5,99); CMII v-*myc* (121,122); OK10 v-*myc* (42); MH2 v-*myc* (33,54,59,89)

[b]All codons from the 416 chicken c-*myc* codons are shown for which the homologous counterparts in at least one of the v-*myc* alleles are changed (as indicated) or deleted (dashes).

[c]CGG:Arg in ref. 5.

[d]AGA:Arg in ref. 5.

[e]CTG:Leu in refs. 33, 54, 89.

[f]GCC:Ala in ref. 89.

[g]AGC:Ser in ref. 89.

for the presumed splice junction was obtained by nucleotide sequence analysis of proviral DNA from a transforming retrovirus that was apparently generated by encapsidation and reverse transcription of MH2 v-*myc* mRNA (89). Analysis revealed precise fusion of the first six *gag* codons to the v-*myc* sequences corresponding to the 5' end of the second exon in c-*myc* (see below). The open reading frame on the MH2 v-*myc* mRNA encodes a 423-amino acid protein (six amino acid residues encoded by *gag*; five encoded by v-*myc* sequences derived from 5' untranslated sequences of the second c-*myc* exon; and 412 encoded by v-*myc* sequences corresponding to the c-*myc* coding domain) with a calculated molecular weight of approximately 46,000 (Fig. 1) (59,89). The translational product was identified in extracts from MH2-transformed cells by immunoprecipitation using antisera against *myc*-specific protein domains. In gel electrophoresis, the protein appears as a characteristic doublet corresponding to apparent molecular weights of 59,000 and 61,000, respectively (p59/61^{v-myc}) (41,54,91). As with all avian and mammalian *myc* protein products, the large discrepancy between calculated and apparent molecular weight of the MH2 v-*myc* gene product is presumably due to unusual structural features of the protein inherent in its primary structure (e.g., the exceptionally high proline content).

The MH2 v-*mil* allele is inserted between the partial *gag* sequences at its 5' end and intron-derived v-*myc* sequences at its 3' end. Comparison of v-*mil* with the chicken c-*mil* gene showed that in the course of the transduction, coding domains derived from 11 exons of the cellular gene were precisely fused (51,55,56,108). The 5' end of v-*mil* is derived from sequences within the coding domain of an exon, and the 3' end corresponds to a position 12 nucleotides downstream of the translational termination codon shared between v-*mil* and c-*mil*. In the MH2 genome, the partial *gag* and the v-*mil* sequences are fused into one large reading frame encoding a 894-amino acid protein (515 amino acid residues encoded by *gag* and 379 encoded by v-*mil*) with a calculated molecular weight of approximately 97,000 (Fig. 1) (59,108). The translational product of this reading frame on genome–sized mRNA was identified in extracts from MH2-transformed cells by immunoprecipitation using antisera against *gag* or *mil* domains (48,90). The *gag-mil* hybrid protein has an apparent molecular weight of 100,000 (p100$^{gag-mil}$). The predicted sequences of MH2 v-*mil* and chicken c-*mil* protein products differ by only five substitutions among the 379 amino acid residues of the shared carboxyl-terminal domains (51). The amino-terminal domain (approximately 270 amino acid residues) of the cellular c-*mil* protein is encoded by 5' c-*mil* sequences that have not been transduced into the genome of MH2 (51,90). In a puzzling contrast to the close proximity of the v-*mil* and v-*myc* alleles in the MH2 genome, the c-*mil* and c-*myc* loci are not physically linked on the chicken genome (55,56,109a).

A strong genetic indication for the oncogenic potential of the MH2 v-*myc* oncogene comes from its close structural relationship to the v-*myc* alleles found as singularly transduced cell-derived inserts in the genomes of MC29, CMII, and OK10, the other members of the MC29 subgroup of avian acute leukemia viruses (9,11–13). Furthermore, analyses of the genetic structures of spontaneous and *in vitro*-constructed mutants of MH2 have provided direct evidence that v-*myc* apparently is the primary oncogenic determinant of MH2. A spontaneous *mil* deletion mutant of MH2, termed MH2D12, and *in vitro*-constructed *mil* deletion mutants all have retained the capacity to transform mass cultures of fibroblasts and to induce focus formation or soft agar colonies of transformed avian embryo cells (7,54,57). These mutants are also still capable of transforming macrophage-like cells in bone marrow cultures (36; see below). Hence, expression of the v-*myc* gene is sufficient and that of the v-*mil* gene not necessary for these activities. The potential of the MH2 v-*myc* allele to act as an autonomously transforming oncogene is further demonstrated by the surprising molecular and biological properties of a spontaneous variant of MH2, termed MH2E21 (Fig. 2). This transforming retrovirus has a remarkably small genome of only 2.3 kilobases and yet is transmissible when supplied with a nondefective helper virus. Complete nucleotide sequence analysis of the proviral DNA from this virus has revealed that it apparently was generated by encapsidation and reverse transcription of the subgenomic MH2 v-*myc* mRNA (89). It encodes a 423-amino acid v-*myc* protein with six *gag* en-

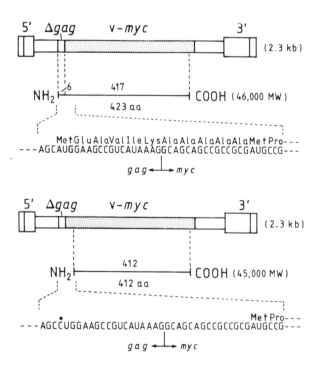

FIG. 2. Genetic structures of MH2 derivatives MH2E21 *(top)* and MH2E21m1 *(bottom)*. Genome-sized mRNAs and their protein products are shown. MH2E21 is a spontaneous variant of MH2 presumably generated by encapsidation and reverse transcription of subgenomic MH2 v-*myc* mRNA (compare Fig. 1.). MH2E21m1 was constructed by *in vitro* mutation of the *gag* translational initiation codon on MH2E21 proviral DNA. The nucleotide substitution is indicated (*).

coded amino acid residues at its amino terminus, indistinguishable from the v-*myc* protein specified by *wt*MH2 (Figs. 1 and 2). Using oligonucleotide-directed mutagenesis, another mutant, termed MH2E21m1, was derived from MH2E21 (89). In this mutant, the translational initiation codon within the *gag* sequences has been mutated, and translation of the MH2E21m1 v-*myc* gene is initiated at the first *myc* AUG codon, which is homologous to that presumably used for the translation of the c-*myc* gene. The 412-amino acid protein product of MH2E21m1 v-*myc* has a calculated molecular weight of approximately 45,000 (Fig. 2), and the protein doublet seen in gel electrophoresis corresponds to an apparent molecular weight of 57,000/59,000 (89). Like MH2E21, MH2E21m1 is capable of transforming avian fibroblasts. Hence, the functional expression of sequences exclusively derived from the c-*myc* coding region is sufficient for cell transformation by the MH2 v-*myc* oncogene. It can be argued that the multiple nucleotide substitutions or deletions within the MH2 v-*myc* allele, compared to its cellular progenitor (Table 1), may be responsible for the oncogenic activation of the gene. However, the other oncogenic v-*myc* alleles contain only a few or even only one mutation, and more important, there is no common mutation found in all v-*myc* alleles (Table 1) (122). Also, *in vitro* replacement of most of the v-*myc* allele of MH2E21 ml by the corresponding CMII v-*myc* sequences has generated a fibroblast-transforming virus with a v-*myc* coding region nearly isogenic with that of the c-*myc* gene (89).

The first genetic indication that v-*mil* may contribute to the oncogenic specificities of MH2 came from the discovery that v-*mil* is closely related to v-*raf* (52), the single oncogene of murine sarcoma virus 3611 (3611-MSV) (97). Nucleotide sequence analyses confirmed that v-*mil* and v-*raf* are derived from cognate cellular genes of avian and mammalian species (59,108). It is surprising that spontaneous or constructed deletion and frame-shift mutants of MH2 lacking a functional v-*myc* allele but retaining a complete v-*mil* allele inefficient in transforming avian fibroblasts (7,57,126). This is in marked contrast to the transforming ability of the murine homolog v-*raf*, which apparently is sufficient for the transformation of mammalian fibroblasts (97,98). It is unknown whether this discrepancy in the oncogenic potential of v-*mil* and v-*raf* is due to the structural differences between the avian and the murine alleles (52,108) or whether it is due to the different environments in avian and mammalian cells, possibly causing different susceptibilities to the oncogene activity. The spontaneous or constructed v-*myc* deletion mutants of MH2 also fail to transform macrophages in bone marrow cultures (36). The only avian cells reported to be affected by these v-*mil*[+]/v-*myc*[−] mutants are chicken neuroretina cells, which are induced to proliferate without apparent transformation on infection by these mutants (7; see below).

Although it is clear from the studies described above that v-*myc* is responsible for the basic oncogenic potential of MH2, additive or complementary function of the v-*myc* and v-*mil* alleles of MH2 has been inferred from several lines of evidence. MH2 was reported to be significantly more oncogenic in infected birds than viruses carrying only v-*myc* (72). Also, natural or constructed v-*mil* deletion mutants of MH2 were shown to be less oncogenic than *wt*MH2 (36), and fibroblasts transformed by v-*mil* deletion mutants or by *wt*MH2 may be differentially affected in certain transformation-associated parameters (54,89). Furthermore, these v-*mil* deletion mutants are capable of transforming macrophages in a bone marrow transformation assay (see above); however, these cells are dependent on the presence of a myelomonocytic growth factor, wheras macrophages transformed by *wt*MH2 are growth factor independent and grow in an autocrine manner (36). The abrogation of growth factor requirement of myeloid cells transformed by v-*myc*- (or v-*myb*) containing viruses can also be achieved by superinfection of these cultures by MH2 (or other viruses containing oncogenes of the *src* family), suggesting that v-*mil* (which is a member of the *src* family; see below) may be responsible for this effect (3). Cooperation or complementation between v-*myc* and v-*mil* has also been suggested as a critical event in the transformation of neuroretina cells. Expression of v-*myc* has no apparent effect on these cells; expression of v-*mil* induces them to proliferate (see above); and concomitant expression of v-*myc* and v-*mil* (such as happens on infection with MH2) leads to cell transformation (7). Similarly, infection with MH2 alters both the differentiated phenotype (e.g., leading to total suppression of collagen synthesis) and the proliferative capacity of definitive chondroblasts, whereas viruses containing only v-*myc* affect only the latter property (4). Constructed murine retroviruses containing both v-*mil*(*raf*) and v-*myc* genes (57) were shown to induce the rapid growth of hematopoietic neoplasms and carcinomas in newborn mice (96), in contrast to the fibrosarcomas induced by 3611-MSV (97,98), and to induce growth factor-independent growth and immortalization of hematopoietic cells *in vitro* (16,95). All these observations suggest that the combination of v-*myc* and v-*mil* on the MH2 genome may enhance the transforming activity and enlarge the oncogenic spectrum of this virus. Based on experiments confirming the autonomous function of MH2 v-*myc* in fibroblast transformation, it has been argued that MH2 behaves like a virus with a single oncogene and that incorporation of v-*mil* could have been an accidental event with no consequences for the transforming (or replicative) capacities of the virus (126). Aside from the possibility that fibroblast transformation may not be the appropriate assay to measure the contribution of v-*mil* to the oncogenic potential of MH2, it appears rather unlikely that such an accidental and irrelevant incorporation would involve a gene, of all genes, which on another occasion (the genesis of 3611-MSV) has been transduced as an active oncogene and which also has been identified in transforming DNA sequences isolated from human cancer cells (32,105). Conversely, the existence, the significance, and the nature of the presumed cooperation or complementation between v-*mil* and v-*myc* can only be assessed when the functions of the oncogene protein products relevant to the induction, maintenance, and progression of the transformed state become known. Nothing is yet known about the critical biochemical functions of v-*myc* and v-*mil* protein products in transformed cells or about the molecular mechanisms leading to cell transformation. There are some preliminary hints at possibly relevant properties of these proteins. The v-*myc* protein products are phosphorylated (14,94) and found predominantely in cell nuclei (1,27,41). Although *myc* protein products bind nonspecifically to DNA *in vitro,* only a minor fraction of these proteins appears to be associated with chromatin structures in intact nuclei (27,29). Based on comparisons of predicted protein sequences (33,108), the *mil(raf)* oncogene is related to the members of the *src* gene family, most of which encode proteins that are associated with tyrosine-specific protein kinase activities. However, phosphorylation of *mil(raf)* gene products *in vivo,* where they are mainly located in the cytoplasm (41), and *in vitro* involves threonine and serine rather than tyrosine residues (94,98,108).

The cotransduction in one retroviral genome of sequences that are not linked on the cellular genome is a puzzling observation. The chicken c-*myc* and c-*mil* loci do not map in proximity to each other, and nucleotide sequence comparison between MH2 proviral DNA and the c-*myc* and c-*mil* loci has failed to reveal any hints (such as limited-sequence homologies) at the mechanism of the actual recombination between these components (51). Hence, it may be difficult to resolve whether MH2 arose by the sequential acquisition of the two cell-derived inserts or whether the c-*myc* and c-*mil* loci had been juxtaposed, possibly by chromosomal translocations or DNA rearrangements prior to their transduction from the tumor cells from which MH2 was isolated.

erb-B and *erb*-A in AEV-R

The genetic structure of AEV-R (10,11,70,119) is shown in Fig. 3. The AEV-R genome contains a 5′ segment of *gag,* a 3′ segment of *env,* and between them the v-*erb*-A and v-*erb*-B alleles. It has been shown that a very short region of *env*-related sequences is interspersed between the two cell-derived inserts (47). At its 5′ end, the v-*erb*-B allele contains a segment apparently derived from c-*erb*-B in-

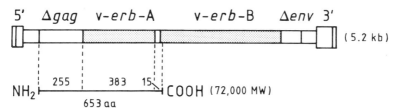

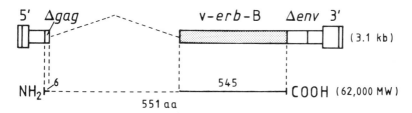

FIG. 3. Genetic structure of avian erythroblastosis virus strain R (AEV-R). Genome-sized and subgenomic mRNAs and their protein products are shown.

tron sequences directly adjacent to the 5' end of an exon, including the splice acceptor site (47). At its 3' end, the junction between v-*erb*-B and *env* sequences apparently corresponds to sequences within a coding exon of c-*erb*-B (81,82). Although only partial nucleotide sequence analyses of the chicken c-*erb*-B locus have so far been reported, it is clear that only a partial complement of the coding region (truncated at both ends) of the cellular gene has been transduced into the genome of AEV-R (81; see below). Nucleotide sequence analyses of the AEV-R v-*erb*-B allele have indicated that it is closely related to the similarly truncated v-*erb*-B allele of AEV-H, another member of the AEV-subgroup of acute leukemia viruses (see below) but that it is distinguished from the homolog in AEV-H by the deletion of 60 codons near and at the 3' end (82,100,125; M. Hayman, *personal communication*). The predicted amino acid sequence of the AEV-H v-*erb*-B protein product differs by only one amino acid exchange from the predicted sequence within the corresponding domain of the c-*erb*-B gene product (81,125). The expression of the AEV-R v-*erb*-B allele is mediated by translation of a subgenomic mRNA species (Fig. 3) that is found in AEV-R-transformed cells in addition to genome-sized mRNA (6) and that is generated by utilization of the standard viral splice donor site (see above) and the c-*erb*-B-derived splice acceptor site (47). The open reading frame on the subgenomic mRNA encodes a 551-amino acid protein (six amino acid residues encoded by *gag,* 545 by v-*erb*-B sequences; the very first out-of-frame *env* codon is the terminator) with a calculated molecular weight of approximately 62,000 (Fig. 3) (82,100,125; M. Hayman, *personal communication*). The translational product of this mRNA was identified by *in vitro* translation of apparently virion-encapsidated mRNA or by immunoprecipitation from extracts of AEV-R-transformed cells using antisera against v-*erb*-B protein domains (44,92). The primary translational product with an apparent molecular weight of 62,000 (p62[v-*erb*-B]) is subsequently processed into a plasma membrane glycoprotein with an apparent molecular weight of 74,000 (gp74[v-*erb*-B]) (43). The 5' border of the v-*erb*-A allele in AEV-R is precisely defined by its fusion with conserved *gag* sequences (23). Between the 3' end of v-*erb*-A and the 5' end of v-*erb*-B (unambiguously defined by comparison with the nucleotide sequence of chicken c-*erb*-B) is a stretch of 30 nucleotides that shares a significant (82%) sequence homology with a segment of avian retroviral *env* genes (47). The localization of the exact 3' border of v-*erb*-A and a more definitive identification of viral sequences interspersed between v-*erb*-A and v-*erb*-B will depend on nucleotide sequence analysis of the corresponding region of the chicken c-*erb*-A locus. Expression of the v-*erb*-A allele is mediated by translation of genome-sized mRNA (Fig. 3). The open reading frame on this mRNA encodes a 653-amino acid protein (255 amino acid residues encoded by *gag;* 383 encoded by v-*erb*-A sequences; and 15 encoded by the *env*-related sequences and by intron-derived v-*erb*-B sequences) with a calculated molecular weight of approximately 72,000 (Fig. 3) (23). Since the open reading frame extends throughout the v-*erb*-A allele, the transduction of the c-*erb*-A gene apparently involved truncation of the coding region. The translational product of genome-sized AEV-R mRNA was identified as a protein with an apparent molecular weight of 75,000 (p75$^{gag\text{-}erb\text{-}A}$) by immunoprecipitation from extracts of AEV-R-transformed cells using antisera against *gag* proteins (45).

There is clear evidence from the analyses of conditional and nonconditional mutants of AEV strains that v-*erb*-B is the dominant oncogenic determinant of these viruses. This is in fact most directly demonstrated by the genetic structure of the independently isolated strain AEV-H, which contains in its genome a v-*erb*-B allele as the only cell-derived insert (125). Like AEV-R, AEV-H induces both erythroblastosis and sarcoma in infected birds, indicating that v-*erb*-A is not necessary and that v-*erb*-B is necessary and possibly sufficient for the induction and maintenance of erythroid and fibroblastic cell transformation. The biological properties of mutants constructed *in vitro* by the introduction of large-deletion or frame-shift mutations in the v-*erb*-A or the v-*erb*-B allele of AEV-R proviral DNA are consistant with the notion that the main transforming potential is encoded by v-*erb*-B (31,102,103). Mutations in the v-*erb*-B allele, except when they are very close to the 3' end, abolish all cell-transforming capacities of AEV-R. In contrast, mutants that have suffered large deletions in the *gag*-v-*erb*-A domain are still capable of transforming fibroblasts and erythroid cells *in vitro,* and some of them induce erythroid leukemia and sarcomas in chickens. Furthermore, all characterized conditional mutants of AEV-R are temperature sensitive for the transformation of both erythroid cells and fibroblasts (87). Hence, disregarding the unlikely possibility that all these mutants contain multiple lesions, their phenotype confirms that the basic capacity of AEV-R for both fibroblastic and erythroid cell transformation is encoded by one gene, i.e., the v-*erb*-B allele (see above).

Since v-*erb*-A of AEV-R is the only known transduced allele of the c-*erb*-A gene and since it is accompanied by the bona fide oncogenic v-*erb*-B allele, there is no straightforward genetic argument in favor of its oncogenic potential, as can be put forward for the multiply transduced *myc, mil,* and *erb*-B oncogenes (see above). Furthermore, the v-*erb*-A^{+}/v-*erb*-B^{-} mutants described above lack any apparent transforming activity. There is evidence, however, that the v-*erb*-A allele contributes to the oncogenic specificities of AEV-R. Erythroblasts transformed by v-*erb*-A^{-}/v-*erb*-B^{+} mutants are not as tightly blocked in their differentiation pathway as those transformed by *wt*AEV-R, and they also require specific factors for growth in culture. Hence, *wt*AEV-R-transformed erythroblasts with their greater proliferation rate, total loss of differentiation capacity, and factor-independent growth may represent a more advanced stage of leukemogenicity, possibly induced by the concomitant expression of the v-*erb*-A and v-*erb*-B alleles of AEV-R (35). Again, the nature of such a presumed cooperation can only be assessed unequivocally, when the biochemical functions of v-*erb*-A and v-*erb*-B protein products in transformed cells become known. Attempts to unveil the molecular mechanisms of v-*erb*-B-induced cell transformation are based on the discoveries of structural homology of the v-*erb*-B protein with gene products of the *src* family of oncogenes (125) and of its strikingly close relationship to the transmembrane and intracellular domains of the human epidermal growth factor (EGF) receptor (24,114). Concordantly, the v-*erb*-B protein product was found to be associated with tyrosine-specific protein kinase activity (34,69) and to be inserted into the plasma membrane (43,100). If v-*erb*-B is indeed derived from a structural and functional avian homolog of the EGF receptor gene, it remains to be elucidated how expression of extensively truncated receptor molecules, lacking most of their ligand binding domain, leads to cell transformation. Notably, insertion mutagenesis of the chicken c-*erb*-B locus observed in erythroblastosis induced by nondefective retroviruses without oncogenes involves truncations of the gene similar to those observed in the transduced alleles (81). The biochemical function specified by the v-*erb*-A allele is unknown. The p75$^{gag-erb-A}$ protein is a phosphoprotein found predominantly in the cytoplasm (1,14,44). It has been reported that the predicted amino acid sequence of the carboxyl-terminal domain of the v-*erb*-A encoded region of the p75 hybrid protein is distantly related to the sequences of carbonic anhydrases (23). There is no evidence that this distant homology extends to any functional properties. Presumably more significant homologies have recently been found between the amino acid sequence of the v-*erb*-A protein product and those of human steroid receptors (37,38,124).

As has been discussed above for the cotransduction of c-*myc* and c-*mil* in the genesis of MH2, there is no clue as to the mechanism by which AEV-R acquired sequences of two unlinked cellular loci. The chicken c-*erb*-B locus is located on a large chromosome, and the c-*erb*-A locus maps to a microchromosome (110). If sequence analysis of the c-*erb*-A locus will indeed prove that the sequences interspersed between v-*erb*-A and v-*erb*-B (Fig. 3) are of viral origin, then a sequential incorporation of the two inserts may have occured in the evolution of AEV-R.

COTRANSDUCED SEQUENCES ENCODING A SINGLE HYBRID PROTEIN

There are several retroviral isolates specifying single transforming proteins that are encoded by sequences derived from more than one cellular locus: (a) avian erythroblastosis (myeloblastosis) virus E26, a member of the AMV subgroup (defined by shared v-*myb* oncogenes) of avian acute leukemia viruses (9,12,13); (b) the Gardner-Rasheed feline sarcoma virus (GR-FeSV) (79,80); (c) the FBR murine osteosarcoma virus (FBR-MSV) (22,115); and (d) Rous sarcoma virus (RSV) (101,111). In every case, there is direct evidence for the oncogenic potential of one of the two cell-derived components, either based on the observation of multiple transduction of the homologous cellular gene in independent retroviral isolates or on extensive genetic analyses (for RSV). The second component encodes either substantial domains of the hybrid proteins (in E26 and GR-FeSV) or only a few carboxyl-terminal amino acid residues (in FBR-MSV and RSV). The latter genetic arrangement may also be true for the genome of the McDonough strain of feline sarcoma virus carrying the v-*fms* oncogene. It was recently shown that the carboxy-terminal 11 amino acid residues of the v-*fms* protein product are encoded by sequences apparently neither derived from c-*fms* nor from virion genes (20). There is still very little knowledge about the functional significance and consequences of these peculiar arrangements of various cell-derived sequences fused in single reading frames.

myb and *ets* in E26

The genetic structure of E26 (15,71,84) is depicted in Fig. 4. The E26 genome contains a 5' complement of *gag* and a 3' complement of *env,* but no *pol* sequences. The v-*myb* and v-*ets* alleles are inserted next to each other, between the partial *gag* and *env* sequences with no viral sequences interspersed between the cell-derived inserts. The E26 v-*myb* allele represents a truncated form of the chicken c-*myb* coding region, which extends both 5' and 3' of the domain defined by the transduced complement. Within the shared domains, the predicted sequences of E26 v-*myb* and chicken c-*myb* protein products differ by a single amino acid exchange (64,85). The structural relationship between E26 v-*ets* and cellular c-*ets* alleles is surprisingly complex: v-*ets* coding domains may be derived from as much as three different chicken loci, from which at least two, however, appear to be physically linked (J. Ghysdael and D. Stehelin, *personal communication*), and in man, two distinct loci containing sequences homologous to different v-*ets* domains were identified on two different chromosomes (122a). The v-*myb* and v-*ets* alleles of E26 are expressed in one translational unit generated by the fusion of *gag, myb,* and *ets* reading frames. The open reading frame on genome-sized mRNA encodes a 1,046-amino acid protein (272 amino acid residues encoded by *gag*; 283 by v-*myb*; and 491 by v-*ets*) with a calculated molecular weight of approximately 115,000 (Fig. 4) (84,85). The translational product of this mRNA was identified in E26-transformed cells as a protein of apparent molecular weight 135,000 (p135$^{gag\text{-}myb\text{-}ets}$) by immunoprecipitation from cellular extracts using antisera against *gag* proteins (15). The genetic origin of the protein was confirmed by tryptic peptide analysis and by immunoprecipitation using antisera specific for *myb* protein domains (63). Although v-*myb* and v-*ets* sequences are so closely linked in the E26 genome and are even cotranslated, their cellular progenitors do not map in close proximity on the chicken genome (71,84,85,109a).

The most straightforward indication for the oncogenic potential of the E26 v-*myb* allele comes from its close structural relationship to the v-*myb* allele of

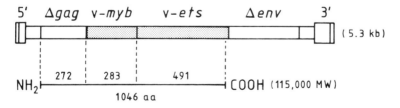

FIG. 4. Genetic structure of avian erythroblastosis (myeloblastosis) virus E26. Genome-size mRNA and its protein product are shown.

avian myeloblastosis virus (AMV), which contains only this single cell-derived insert (25,64). The v-*myb* allele of AMV (which also represents a truncated form of c-*myb*) differs from that of E26 mainly by the presence of intron-derived sequences and nine additional codons at the 5' end and of 79 additional codons at the 3' end (64,85). Also, expression of the AMV v-*myb* allele is mediated by the translation of a subgenomic mRNA yielding a protein with only a few terminal amino acid residues encoded by virion gene sequences (62,64,65). Although AMV and E26 contain oncogenes derived from a common progenitor, they exhibit pronounced differences in their pathogenic properties. AMV exclusively induces myeloblastosis in infected chickens, whereas E26 predominantly causes erythroblastosis or mixed erythroid (myeloid) leukemias (77,107). Furthermore, E26 induces transformation of both erythroid and myeloid cells in bone marrow cultures and of fibroblasts in some avian species, whereas AMV exclusively transforms cells of the myeloid lineage (93). It has not yet been analyzed in a systematic fashion whether the differences in structure and mode of expression between the two v-*myb* alleles or the addition of the v-*ets* allele in E26 or both are responsible for the different pathogenic activities of these viruses. It is conceivable that the v-*ets*-encoded domain of the single *gag-myb-ets* protein product of the E26 genome may either modulate the function of the v-*myb*-encoded domain or add new functional properties to the protein, leading to the broadening of the oncogenic spectrum of E26 compared to that of AMV. Conditional mutants of E26 have been described that are temperature sensitive in their ability to transform myeloid cells while retaining the capacity to transform erythroid cells at the nonpermissive temperature (8). This could imply, but is not proven, that the phenotype of this mutants reflects the presence of independent functional domains on the single-protein product of E26. Of course, there is still no evidence that *ets* has oncogenic potential on its own, particularly since it has not been found in any other retroviral isolate. The biochemical functions of v-*myb* and v-*ets* protein products in transformed cells are unknown. The p135$^{gag-myb-ets}$ protein is phosphorylated and is found predominantly in the nuclei of transformed cells (15,66).

The chicken c-*myb* and c-*ets* loci do not map in close proximity to each other (see above), and it is entirely unclear how a single retroviral genome could have acquired sequences from two unlinked cellular genes whose coding regions are even fused in a single reading frame and expressed as a hybrid polyprotein as a result of the cotransduction. It is interesting to note that there have been reports on cellular oncogenes being fused with genes from different chromosomes, very similar to the fusion of *myb* and *ets* in the E26 genome but without any apparent involvement of retroviral transduction. The Philadelphia chromosome, a chromosomal abnormality observed in the leukemic cells of more than 90% of patients with chronic myeloid leukemia, is generated by a reciprocal translocation between chromosomes 9 and 22. As a consequence of the translocation, the c-*abl* oncogene from chromosome 9 and the *bcr* locus on chromosome 22 are fused in such a way that they are transcribed into a chimeric mRNA encoding a hybrid polyprotein with presumably novel and possibly oncogenic biochemical functions, compared to the normal c-*abl* gene product (2,39,46,68,106). Furthermore, a human onco-gene (termed *onc*D or *trk*) isolated from a colon carcinoma was shown to be gener-ated by the juxtaposition and in-frame fusion of truncated forms of genes encoding tropomyosin and a putative transmembrane receptor with homology to protein ty-rosine kinases, respectively (73).

fgr and Actin in GR-FeSV

The genetic structure of GR-FeSV (79,80) is shown in Fig. 5. The viral genome contains partial complements of the *gag* and *env* genes, but no *pol* sequences. The cell-derived sequences inserted between the partial virion genes are apparently de-rived from two different cellular loci, one representing the cat γ-actin gene, and the other, c-*fgr*, representing a gene closely related to members of the *src* family of oncogenes. Although the cat γ-actin and c-*fgr* genes have not yet been exten-sively characterized, the two cell-derived components in the GR-FeSV genome can be clearly identified by their extensive homologies to known genes from dif-ferent species. The v-γ-actin encoded protein sequences are virtually identical with those of the amino-terminal third of the cytoplasmic γ-actins from various mam-malian species (79,83,117). The other insert, v-*fgr*, encodes protein sequences with a striking homology to those encoded by the *yes* oncogene, a member of the *src* family transduced in the genome of avian sarcoma virus Y73 (60,79). This does not imply, however, that the cat c-*fgr* and the chicken c-*yes* genes are cognate genes, since it has been demonstrated that c-*src*, c-*yes*, and c-*fgr* are related, but distinct, loci in man and that human c-*fgr* is identical with the independently de-fined human c-*src*-2 locus (113). The v-γ-actin and v-*fgr* alleles fo GR-FeSV are expressed in one translational unit generated by the fusion of *gag*, actin, and *fgr* reading frames. The open reading frame on genome-sized mRNA encodes a 663-amino acid protein (118 amino acid residues encoded by *gag*; 22 encoded by se-quences possibly derived from the 5′ noncoding region of the cat γ-actin gene; 128 encoded by sequences with homology to the mammalian γ-actin genes; 390 encoded by v-*fgr*; and five encoded by out-of-frame *env* sequences) with a calcu-

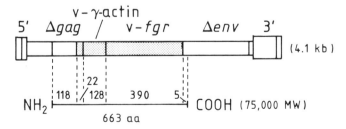

FIG. 5. Genetic structure of Gardner-Rasheed feline sarcoma virus (GR-FeSV). Genome-sized mRNA and its protein product are shown. (Note, that the prefix v- is used to distinguish any transduced sequence in a retroviral genome from its cellular counterpart.)

lated molecular weight of approximately 75,000 (Fig. 5) (79). The corresponding translational product was identified in GR-FeSV-transformed cells by immunoprecipitation using antisera against *gag* proteins as a protein with an apparent molecular weight of 70,000 (p70$^{gag\text{-}actin\text{-}fgr}$) (78,80).

It is reasonable to assume that the basic oncogenic potential of GR-FeSV is due to the functional expression of its v-*fgr* allele. This is mainly based on the close structural relationship of v-*fgr* to oncogenes belonging to the *src* family. Concordantly, the p70$^{gag\text{-}actin\text{-}fgr}$ gene product was shown to be associated with tyrosine-specific protein kinase activity (78). Naturally, it would be important to know whether the amino-terminal actin protein sequences in the GR-FeSV protein product are of any functional significance. Actins constitute a family of highly conserved proteins found in all eukaryotic cells, and their cytoplasmic forms participate in a variety of functions related to cell motility and cytoskeleton structure. Although it is intriguing to find a partial complement of such a gene in the genome of a highly oncogenic virus, there is no evidence that mutant actin genes have autonomous oncogenic potential and they have not been found in other retroviral isolates. There have been no reports on the relative locations of γ-actin and c-*fgr* genes on the cat genome, but in man they appear not to be closely linked (113). Hence, the genesis of GR-FeSV presumably also involved cotransduction of unlinked cellular loci.

fos and *fox* in FBR-MSV

The genetic structure of FBR-MSV (22,115) is depicted in Fig. 6. The genome contains a 5' segment of *gag* and a very small 3' remnant of the *env* gene. Inserted between these partial virion genes are two cell-derived inserts, v-*fos* and v-*fox,* which are directly adjacent to each other with no viral sequences interspersed. Nucleotide sequence comparison has revealed that the FBR-MSV v-*fos* allele represents a truncated form of the mouse c-*fos* coding region, with codons deleted from both termini and from internal positions (115,116). The structural relationship of the v-*fox* allele to its cellular progenitor has not yet been described. The v-*fos* allele is expressed by translation of a fused *gag-fos* reading frame that terminates within the v-*fox* sequences shortly after the *fos-fox* junction. This reading frame on genome-sized mRNA encodes a 554-amino acid protein (310 amino acid resi-

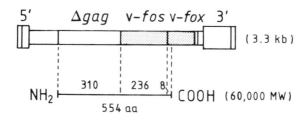

FIG. 6. Genetic structure of FBR murine osteosarcoma virus (FBR-MSV). Genome-size mRNA and its protein product are shown.

dues encoded by *gag;* 236 encoded by v-*fos;* and eight encoded by v-*fox*) with a calculated molecular weight of approximately 60,000 (Fig. 6) (115). The corresponding translational product was identified by immunoprecipitation from extracts of FBR-MSV-transformed cells as a protein with an apparent molecular weight of 75,000 (p75$^{gag\text{-}fos}$) (22). As with *myc* protein products (see above), the large discrepancy between calculated and apparent molecular weight of *fos* protein products may be due to unusual amino acid composition (115). The v-*fox* allele contains no significant open reading frame, and it is not known whether the eight codons and the termination signal used for the synthesis of the p75 protein are derived from a putative c-*fox* coding region. Nucleotide sequence analysis of the mouse c-*fox* locus, for which transcripts have been identified in normal mouse cells (115), is required to resolve this issue.

Genetic indication for the oncogenic potential of the FBR-MSV v-*fos* allele comes from its close relationship to the v-*fos* allele identified in another strain of murine osteosarcoma virus, termed FBJ-MSV (115,116). The v-*fos* allele of FBJ-MSV is the only cell-derived insert in the genome of this virus. Although the two v-*fos* alleles are closely related and derived from the same cellular progenitor, they are distinguished in structure, mode of gene expression, and relative transforming activity (76,115,116). The FBJ-MSV v-*fos* allele specifies a protein exclusively encoded by c-*fos*-derived sequences; however, although the amino terminus of the v-*fos*-encoded protein is identical to that of the c-*fos* protein product, the carboxyl terminal is modified by a frame-shift deletion in the v-*fos* allele (116). Hence, both oncogenic mutant alleles of c-*fos* (i.e., the transduced v-*fos* alleles), encode proteins with modified carboxyl terminals. If this modification is indeed involved in the activation of the oncogenic potential of the *fos* gene, it certainly is not specific in its requirements for the substituted sequences, and it provides no evidence for any specific functional role of the v-*fox* sequences in the FBR-MSV genome. Furthermore, it has been demonstrated that the unmodified c-*fos* protein product is capable of transforming fibroblasts, provided that the c-*fos* gene is linked to retroviral long-terminal-repeat sequences and that the 3′ noncoding region is interrupted (74,75). Hence, the functional significance of the structural changes of v-*fos* protein products is not clear and may only be assessed when the biochemical functions of these proteins in transformed cells, where they are mainly located in the nucleus (21), become known.

src and *src′* in RSV

The genetic structure of nondefective RSV (40,101,111,120) containing all three replicative genes and the v-*src* oncogene is shown in Fig. 7. It is interesting to note that it has been suggested that the original isolate of RSV was replication defective and that the transduction of *src* occurred at the expense of replicative genes of the transducing virus (26), because it has been observed for all other cases of oncogene transduction (13,118). Nondefective RSV would then have been generated during subsequent recombination between the replication-defective RSV and a nondefective helper virus (26). The 5′ end of the v-*src* allele corresponds to

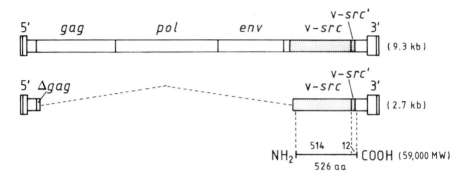

FIG. 7. Genetic structure of avian Rous sarcoma virus (RSV). Genomic RNA and the 2.7-kb subgenomic mRNA and its protein product are shown.

sequences upstream of the chicken c-*src* coding region, including a splice acceptor signal. Sequences derived from a 5′ noncoding exon and from 11 coding exons of c-*src* have been precisely fused in the generation of v-*src,* and the predicted amino acid sequences of the v-*src* and c-*src* protein products differ only by single amino acid exchanges (between eight and 19 of the 514 amino acids of the shared domain, depending on the strain of RSV analyzed) and by the replacement of 19 amino acids at the carboxyl terminal of the c-*src* protein by a different sequence of 12 amino acids at the carboxyl terminals of v-*src* protein products (101,111). The carboxyl-terminal amino acids of v-*src* protein products are encoded by sequences derived from a cellular locus (c-*src′*) located approximately 900 nucleotides downstream of the c-*src* translational termination codon and by viral sequences that also provide the termination codon for the v-*src* protein synthesis. The cellular c-*src* mRNA does not include sequences derived from c-*src′* (111). Expression of the v-*src* allele is mediated by translation of a subgenomic mRNA that is generated from genomic RNA by utilization of the standard viral splice donor site and the c-*src*-derived splice acceptor site (101,111). The open reading frame on this mRNA encodes a 526-amino acid protein (514 amino acid residues encoded by v-*src* and 12 encoded by v-*src′* and viral sequences) with a calculated molecular weight of approximately 59,000 (Fig. 7) (101,111). The corresponding translational product was identified by immunoprecipitation (using antisera from animals bearing RSV-induced tumors) from extracts of RSV-transformed cells as a protein with an apparent molecular weight of 60,000 (p60[v-src]) (17).

The oncogenic potential of the v-*src* oncogene, among all oncogenes, has been established most rigorously by extensive genetic analyses (40,120). Recent efforts have focused on the identification of possibly significant changes in structure and expression between c-*src* and v-*src* that render the transduced allele oncogenic. Expression of an unaltered c-*src* protein product at elevated levels does not lead to any overt cell transformation. This was demonstrated by the introduction into cultured cells of DNA from c-*src*-containing expression plasmids or from RSV constructs in which the entire v-*src* allele was replaced by c-*src*. The recipient cells contained high amounts of the c-*src* protein product (equal to or even higher than those of the v-*src* protein in RSV-transformed cells), and yet these cells remained essentially untransformed (50,88,104). It has been argued that the most obvious structural change at the carboxyl terminals of v-*src* protein products may be essential for the activation of their oncogenic function (19,88,104,124a). On the other hand, RSV constructs in which either the 5′ or the 3′ domain of v-*src* is replaced with the corresponding c-*src* sequences are still transforming, indicating that v-*src* alleles contain at least two mutations, either of which is sufficient to activate oncogenic function (50). Hence, the carboxyl-terminal modification appears not to be an absolute requirement for the activation of the basic transforming activity of v-*src* proteins, and there is no evidence that the c-*src*′-derived sequences confer any specific properties to the protein encoded by the v-*src*/v-*src*′ translational unit. Nevertheless, all these experiments indicate that some qualitative changes in gene function are at the roots of oncogenic activation of the *src* gene, although an interplay between qualitative and quantitative modification of gene function may still be necessary for full oncogenicity. Both c-*src* and v-*src* protein products exhibit *in vitro* tyrosine-specific protein kinase activity, contain myristic acid covalently bound at their amino terminals, and are associated with the plasma membrane in normal and transformed cells, respectively (49).

The cotransduction of c-*src* and c-*src*′ sequences in the RSV genome differs from the cases described in the previous sections in at least two respects. First, c-*src* and c-*src*′ map in close proximity to each other on the chicken genome. Second, nucleotide sequence comparisons among v-*src*, c-*src*, and c-*src*′ have revealed structural features that could explain how the transduction was achieved. The c-*src* and c-*src*′ loci share short homologous sequence elements precisely at the positions corresponding to the *src*/*src*′ junction in RSV v-*src*. Similarly, c-*src*′ and 3′ noncoding viral sequences of avian nondefective helper viruses share homologous segments at the positions corresponding to the *src*′/viral junction in the RSV genome (26,111). These limited regions of homology presumably facilitated the recombination among the three components: c-*src*, c-*src*′, and the transducing virus. Hence, the critical role of c-*src*′ in the evolution of the active v-*src* oncogene may have been to aid in the transduction of the gene rather than to modify its function. Conversely, the disruption of the 3′ end of the c-*src* gene by a recombination with c-*src*′ could have been the first step in its oncogenic activation.

SUMMARY

Biochemical and genetic analyses of genome structure and gene expression have revealed that several highly oncogenic retroviruses contain in their genomes protein-coding nucleotide sequences that are derived from more than one cellular locus. The basic observations are the following:

1. The genomes of MH2 and AEV-R each contain two cell-derived inserts that are expressed as separate protein products by translation of different mRNA spe-

cies. Both protein products are encoded by sequences derived from authentic coding domains of cellular genes.

2. The genomes of E26, GR-FeSV, FBR-MSV, and RSV each contain two cell-derived inserts that are expressed as a hybrid protein by translation of a fused reading frame on a single mRNA species. On E26 and GR-FeSV mRNAs, both cell-derived components contribute substantial complements derived from authentic cellular coding domains to the translational unit encoding the hybrid polyprotein. On FBR-MSV and RSV mRNAs, only one of the two cell-derived inserts provides a substantial and authentic coding region, whereas the other contributes only a few terminal codons, which have not been shown to be derived from coding domains of cellular genes.

3. In all cases of cotransduction, one of the two inserts in the viral genome, and in one case (MH2), each of them, is derived from a cellular gene (protooncogene) whose oncogenic potential has been unambiguously demonstrated by the identification of autonomously oncogenic mutant alleles.

4. For MH2, AEV-R, and E26, an enhancement of oncogenic activity or expansion of the oncogenic spectrum has been observed in comparison to other retroviral isolates or mutants, which carry only one of the respective cell-derived inserts in their genomes.

5. In all but one case (RSV), the cotransduced sequences in retroviral genomes are derived from distant cellular loci. Cotransduction of unlinked cellular genes may have been preceded by chromosomal translocations, although independent sequential recombinations between the transducing virus and cellular loci are also conceivable.

ACKNOWLEDGMENTS

I thank Hans W. Jansen and Tilo Patschinsky for many stimulating discussions and Birgit Schroeer and Christiane Trachmann for excellent assistance with experimental work. Work in my laboratory has been supported by the Max-Planck-Gesellschaft, by the Deutsche Forschungsgemeinschaft, and by the Fonds der Chemischen Industrie.

REFERENCES

1. Abrams, H.D., Rohrschneider, L.R., and Eisenman, R.N. (1982): Nuclear location of the putative transforming protein of avian myelocytomatosis virus. *Cell, 29:*427–439.
2. Adams, J.M. (1985): Oncogene activation by fusion of chromosomes in leukaemia. *Nature,* 315:542–543.
3. Adkins, B., Leutz, A., and Graf, T. (1984): Autocrine growth induced by *src*-related oncogenes in transformed chicken myeloid cells. *Cell,* 39:439–445.
4. Alema, S., Tato, F., and Boettiger, D. (1985): *myc* and *src* Oncogenes have complementary effects on cell proliferation and expression of specific extracellular matrix components in definitive chondroblasts. *Mol. Cell. Biol.,* 5:538–544.
5. Alitalo, K., Bishop, J.M., Smith, D.H., Chen, E.Y., Colby, W.W., and Levinson, A.D.

(1983): Nucleotide sequence of the v-*myc* oncogene of avian retrovirus MC29. *Proc. Natl. Acad. Sci. U.S.A.*, 80:100–104.

6. Anderson, S.M., Hayward, W.S., Neel, B.G., and Hanafusa, H. (1980): Avian erythroblastosis virus produces two mRNAs. *J. Virol.*, 36:676–683.

7. Bechade, C., Calothy, G., Pessac, B., Martin, P., Coll, J., Denhez, F., Saule, S., Ghysdael, J., and Stehelin, D. (1985): Induction of proliferation or transformation of neuroretina cells by the *mil* and *myc* viral oncogenes. *Nature*, 316:559–562.

8. Beug, H., Leutz, A., Kahn, P., and Graf, T. (1984): *ts* Mutants of E26 leukemia virus allow transformed myeloblasts, but not erythroblasts or fibroblasts, to differentiate at the nonpermissive temperature. *Cell*, 39:579–588.

9. Bister, K. (1984): Molecular biology of avian acute leukaemia viruses. In: *Mechanisms of Viral Leukaemogenesis*, edited by J.M. Goldman, and J.O. Jarrett, pp. 38–63. Churchill Livingstone, Edinburgh.

10. Bister, K., and Duesberg, P.H. (1979): Structure and specific sequences of avian erythroblastosis virus RNA: Evidence for multiple classes of transforming genes among avian tumor viruses. *Proc. Natl. Acad. Sci. U.S.A.*, 76:5023–5027.

11. Bister, K., and Duesberg, P.H. (1980): Genetic structure of avian acute leukemia viruses. *Cold Spring Harbor Symp. Quant. Biol.*, 44:801–822.

12. Bister, K., and Duesberg, P.H. (1982): Genetic structure and transforming genes of avian retroviruses. In: *Advances in Viral Oncology, Vol. 1*, edited by G. Klein, pp. 3–42. Raven Press, New York.

13. Bister, K., and Jansen, H.W. (1986): Oncogenes in retroviruses and cells: Biochemistry and molecular genetics. *Adv. Cancer Res.*, 47:99–188.

14. Bister, K., Lee, W.-H., and Duesberg, P.H. (1980): Phosphorylation of the nonstructural proteins encoded by three avian acute leukemia viruses and by avian Fujinami sarcoma virus. *J. Virol.*, 36:617–621.

15. Bister, K., Nunn, M., Moscovici, C., Perbal, B., Baluda, M.A., and Duesberg, P.H. (1982): Acute leukemia viruses E26 and avian myeloblastosis virus have related transformation-specific RNA sequences but different genetic structures, gene products, and oncogenic properties. *Proc. Natl. Acad. Sci. U.S.A.*, 79:3677–3681.

16. Blasi, E., Mathieson, B.J., Varesio, L., Cleveland, J.L., Borchert, P.A., and Rapp, U.R. (1985): Selective immortalization of murine macrophages from fresh bone marrow by a *raf/myc* recombinant murine retrovirus. *Nature*, 318:667–670.

17. Brugge, J.S., and Erikson, R.L. (1977): Identification of a transformation-specific antigen induced by an avian sarcoma virus. *Nature*, 269:346–348.

18. Coll, J., Righi, M., de Taisne, C., Dissous, C., Gegonne, A., and Stehelin, D. (1983): Molecular cloning of the avian acute transforming retrovirus MH2 reveals a novel cell-derived sequence (v-*mil*) in addition to the *myc* oncogene. *EMBO J.*, 2:2189–2194.

19. Cooper, J.A., Gould, K.L., Cartwright, C.A., and Hunter, T. (1986): Tyr^{527} is phosphorylated in pp60^{c-src}: Implications for regulation. *Science*, 231:1431–1433.

20. Coussens, L., Van Beveren, C., Smith, D., Chen, E., Mitchell, R.L., Isacke, C.M., Verma, I.M., and Ullrich, A. (1986): Structural alteration of viral homologue of receptor proto-oncogene *fms* at carboxyl terminus. *Nature*, 320:277–280.

21. Curran, T., Miller, A.D., Zokas, L., and Verma, I.M. (1984): Viral and cellular *fos* proteins: A comparative analysis. *Cell*, 36:259–268.

22. Curran, T., and Verma, I.M. (1984): FBR murine osteosarcoma virus. I. Molecular analysis and characterization of a 75,000-Da *gag-fos* fusion protein. *Virology*, 135:218–228.

23. Debuire, B., Henry, C., Benaissa, M., Biserte, G., Claverie, J.M., Saule, S., Martin, P., and Stehelin, D. (1984): Sequencing of the *erb*A gene of avian erythroblastosis virus reveals a new type of oncogene. *Science*, 224:1456–1459.

24. Downward, J., Yarden, Y., Mayes, E., Srace, G., Totty, N., Stockwell, P., Ullrich, A., Schlessinger, J., and Waterfield, M.D. (1984): Close similarity of epidermal growth factor receptor and v-*erb*-B oncogene protein sequences. *Nature*, 307:521–527.

25. Duesberg, P.H., Bister, K., and Moscovici, C. (1980): Genetic structure of avian myeloblastosis virus, released from transformed myeloblasts as a defective virus particle. *Proc. Natl. Acad. Sci. U.S.A.*, 77:5120–5124.

26. Dutta, A., Wang, L.-H., Hanafusa, T., and Hanafusa, H. (1985): Partial nucleotide sequence of Rous sarcoma virus-29 provides evidence that the original Rous sarcoma virus was replication defective. *J. Virol.*, 55:728–735.

27. Eisenman, R.N., Tachibana, C.Y., Abrams, H.D., and Hann, S.R. (1985): v-*myc*- and c-*myc*-encoded proteins are associated with the nuclear matrix. *Mol. Cell. Biol.,* 5:114–126.
28. Ellis, R.W., Lowy, D.R., and Scholnick, E.M. (1982): The viral and cellular p21 *(ras)* gene family. In: *Advances in Viral Oncology, Vol. 1,* edited by G. Klein, pp. 107–126. Raven Press, New York.
29. Evan, G.I., and Hancock, D.C. (1985): Studies on the interaction of the human c-*myc* protein with cell nuclei: p62^{c-myc} as a member of a discrete subset of nuclear proteins. *Cell,* 43:253–261.
30. Foulds, L. (1958): The natural history of cancer. *J. Chronic Dis.,* 8:2–37.
31. Frykberg, L., Palmieri, S., Beug, H., Graf, T., Hayman, M.J., and Vennström, B. (1983): Transforming capacities of avian erythroblastosis virus mutants deleted in the *erbA* or *erbB* oncogenes. *Cell,* 32:227–238.
32. Fukui, M., Yamamoto, T., Kawai, S., Maruo, K., and Toyoshima, K. (1985): Detection of a *raf*-related and two other transforming DNA sequences in human tumors maintained in nude mice. *Proc. Natl. Acad. Sci. U.S.A.,* 82:5954–5958.
33. Galibert, F., Dupont de Dinechin, S., Righi, M., and Stehelin, D. (1984): The second oncogene *mil* of avian retrovirus MH2 is related to the *src* gene family. *EMBO J.,* 3:1333–1338.
34. Gilmore, T., DeClue, J.E., and Martin, G.S. (1985): Protein phosphorylation at tyrosine is induced by the v-*erbB* gene product *in vivo* and *in vitro. Cell,* 40:609–618.
35. Graf, T., and Beug, H. (1983): Role of the v-*erbA* and v-*erbB* oncogenes of avian erythroblastosis virus in erythroid cell transformation. *Cell,* 34:7–9.
36. Graf, T, von Weizsaecker, F., Grieser, S., Coll, J., Stehelin, D., Patschinsky, T., Bister, K., Bechade, C., Calothy, G., and Leutz, A. (1986): v-*mil* Induces autocrine growth and enhanced tumorigenicity in v-*myc* transformed avian macrophages. *Cell,* 45:357–364.
37. Green, S., Walter, P., Kumar, V., Krust, A., Bornert, J.-M., Argos, P., and Chambon, P. (1986): Human oestrogen receptor cDNA: Sequence, expression and homology to v-*erb*-A. *Nature,* 320:134–139.
38. Greene, G.L., Gilna, P., Waterfield, M., Baker, A., Hort, Y., and Shine, J. (1986): Sequence and expression of human estrogen receptor complementary DNA. *Science,* 231:1150–1154.
39. Grosveld, G., Verwoerd, T., van Agthoven, T., de Klein, A., Ramachandran, K.L., Heisterkamp, N., Stam, K., and Groffen, J. (1986): The chronic myelocytic cell line K562 contains a breakpoint in *bcr* and produces a chimeric *bcr/c-abl* transcript. *Mol. Cell. Biol.,* 6:607–616.
40. Hanafusa, H. (1977): Cell transformation by RNA tumor viruses. In: *Comprehensive Virology, Vol. 10,* edited by H. Fraenkel-Conrat and R.R. Wagner, pp. 401–483. Plenum Press, New York.
41. Hann, S.R., Abrams, H.D., Rohrschneider, L.R., and Eisenman, R.N. (1983): Proteins encoded by v-*myc* and c-*myc* oncogenes: Identification and localization in acute leukemia virus transformants and bursal lymphoma cell lines. *Cell,* 34:789–798.
42. Hayflick, J., Seeburg, P.H., Ohlsson, R., Pfeifer-Ohlsson, S., Watson, D., Papas, T., and Duesberg, P.H. (1985): Nucleotide sequence of two overlapping *myc*-related genes in avian carcinoma virus OK10 and their relation to the *myc* genes of other viruses and the cell. *Proc. Natl. Acad. Sci. U.S.A.,* 82:2718–2722.
43. Hayman, M.J., and Beug, H. (1984): Identification of a form of the avian erythroblastosis virus *erb-B* gene product at the cell surface. *Nature,* 309:460–462.
44. Hayman, M.J., Ramsay, G.M., Savin, K., and Kitchener, G. (1983): Identification and characterization of the avian erythroblastosis virus *erbB* gene product as a membrane glycoprotein. *Cell,* 32:579–588.
45. Hayman, M.J., Royer-Pokora, B., and Graf, T. (1979): Defectiveness of avian erythroblastosis virus: Synthesis of a 75K *gag*-related protein. *Virology,* 92:31–45.
46. Heisterkamp, N., Stam, K., Groffen, J., de Klein, A., and Grosveld, G. (1985): Structural organization of the *bcr* gene and its role in the Ph' translocation. *Nature,* 315:758–761.
47. Henry, C., Coquillaud, M., Saule, S., Stehelin, D., and Debuire, B. (1985): The four C-terminal amino acids of the v-*erbA* polypeptide are encoded by an intronic sequence of the v-*erbB* oncogene. *Virology,* 140:179–182.
48. Hu, S.S.F., Moscovici, C., and Vogt, P.K. (1978): The defectiveness of Mill Hill 2, a carcinoma-inducing avian oncovirus. *Virology,* 89:162–178.
49. Iba, H., Cross, F.R., Garber, E.A., and Hanafusa, H. (1985): Low level of cellular protein phosphorylation by nontransforming overproduced p60^{c-src}. *Mol. Cell. Biol.,* 5:1058–1066.
50. Iba, H., Takeya, T., Cross, F.R., Hanafusa, T., and Hanafusa, H. (1984): Rous sarcoma virus variants that carry the cellular *src* gene instead of the viral *src* gene cannot transform chicken embryo fibroblasts. *Proc. Natl. Acad. Sci. U.S.A.,* 81:4424–4428.

51. Jansen, H.W., and Bister, K. (1985): Nucleotide sequence analysis of the chicken gene c-*mil*, the progenitor of the retroviral oncogene v-*mil*. *Virology*, 143:359–367.
52. Jansen, H.W., Lurz, R., Bister, K., Bonner, T.I., Mark, GE., and Rapp, U.R. (1984): Homologous cell-derived oncogenes in avian carcinoma virus MH2 and murine sarcoma virus 3611. *Nature*, 307:281–284.
53. Jansen, H.W., Patschinsky, T., and Bister, K. (1983): Avian oncovirus MH2: Molecular cloning of proviral DNA and structural analysis of viral RNA and protein. *J. Virol.*, 48:61–73.
54. Jansen, H.W., Patschinsky, T., Walther, N., Lurz, R., and Bister, K. (1985): Molecular and biological properties of MH2D12, a spontaneous *mil* deletion mutant of avian oncovirus MH2. *Virology*, 142:248–262.
55. Jansen, H.W., Rückert, B., Lurz, R., and Bister, K. (1983): Two unrelated cell-derived sequences in the genome of avian leukemia and carcinoma inducing retrovirus MH2. *EMBO J.*, 2:1969–1975.
56. Jansen, H.W., Trachmann, C., and Bister, K. (1984): Structural relationship between the chicken protooncogene c-*mil* and the retroviral oncogene v-*mil*. *Virology*, 137:217–224.
57. Jansen, H.W., Trachmann, C., Patschinsky, T., and Bister, K. (1985): The *mil/raf* and *myc* oncogenes: Molecular cloning and *in vitro* mutagenesis. In: *Modern Trends in Human Leukemia VI*, edited by R. Neth, R.C. Gallo, M. Greaves, and G.Janka, pp. 280–283. Springer Verlag, Berlin-Heidelberg.
58. Kan, N.C., Flordellis, C.S., Garon, C.F., Duesberg, P.H., and Papas, T.S. (1983): Avian carcinoma virus MH2 contains a transformation-specific sequence, *mht*, and shares the *myc* sequence with MC29, CMII, and OK10 viruses. *Proc. Natl. Acad. Sci. U.S.A.*, 80:6566–6570.
59. Kan, N.C., Flordellis, C.S., Mark, G.E., Duesberg, P.H., and Papas, T.S. (1984): Nucleotide sequence of avian carcinoma virus MH2: Two potential *onc* genes, one related to avian virus MC29 and the other related to murine sarcoma virus 3611. *Proc. Natl. Acad. Sci. U.S.A.*, 81:3000–3004.
60. Kitamura, N., Kitamura, A., Toyoshima, K., Hirayama, Y., and Yoshida, M. (1982): Avian sarcoma virus Y73 genome sequence and structural similarity of its transforming gene product to that of Rous sarcoma virus. *Nature*, 297:205–208.
61. Klein, G., and Klein, E. (1985): Evolution of tumours and the impact of molecular oncology. *Nature*, 315:190–195.
62. Klempnauer, K.-H., and Bishop, J.M. (1983): Transduction of c-*myb* into avian myeloblastosis virus: Locating points of recombination within the cellular gene. *J. Virol.*, 48:565–572.
63. Klempnauer, K.-H., and Bishop, J.M. (1984): Neoplastic transformation by E26 leukemia virus is mediated by a single protein containing domains of *gag* and *myb* genes. *J. Virol.*, 50:280–283.
64. Klempnauer, K.-H., Gonda, T.J., and Bishop, J.M. (1982): Nucleotide sequence of the retroviral leukemia gene v-*myb* and its cellular progenitor c-*myb*: The architecture of a transduced oncogene. *Cell*, 31:453–463.
65. Klempnauer, K.-H., Ramsay, G., Bishop, J.M., Moscovici, G.M., Moscovici, C., McGrath, J.P., and Levinson, A.D. (1983): The product of the retroviral transforming gene v-*myb* is a truncated version of the protein encoded by the cellular oncogene c-*myb*. *Cell*, 33:345–355.
66. Klempnauer, K.-H., Symonds, G., Evan, G.I., and Bishop, J.M. (1984): Subcellular localization of proteins encoded by oncogenes of avian myeloblastosis virus and avian leukemia virus E26 and by the chicken c-*myb* gene. *Cell*, 37:537–547.
67. Knudson, A.G. (1973): Mutation and human cancer. *Adv. Cancer Res.*, 17:317–352.
68. Konopka, J.B., Watanabe, S.M., Singer, J.W., Collins, S.J., and Witte, O.N. (1985): Cell lines and clinical isolates derived from Ph'-positive chronic myelogenous leukemia patients express c-*abl* proteins with a common structural alteration. *Proc. Natl. Acad. Sci. U.S.A.*, 82:1810–1814.
69. Kris, R.M., Lax, I., Gullick, W., Waterfield, M.D., Ullrich, A., Fridkin, M., and Schlessinger, J. (1985): Antibodies against a synthetic peptide as a probe for the kinase activity of the avian EGF receptor and v-*erbB* protein. *Cell*, 40:619–625.
70. Lai, M.M.C., Hu, S.S.F., and Vogt, P.K. (1979): Avian erythroblastosis virus: Transformation-specific sequences form a contiguous segment of 3.25 kb located in the middle of the 6-kb genome. *Virology*, 97:366–377.
71. Leprince, D., Gegonne, A., Coll, J., de Taisne, C., Schneeberger, A., Lagrou, C., and Stehelin, D. (1983): A putative second cell-derived oncogene of the avian leukaemia retrovirus E26. *Nature*, 306:395–397.
72. Linial, M. (1982): Two retroviruses with similar transforming genes exhibit differences in transforming potential. *Virology*, 119:382–391.

73. Martin-Zanca, D., Hughes, S.H., and Barbacid, M. (1986): A human oncogene formed by the fusion of truncated tropomyosin and protein tyrosine kinase sequences. *Nature*, 319:743–748.
74. Meijlink, F., Curran, T., Miller, A.D., and Verma, I.M. (1985): Removal of a 67-base-pair sequence in the noncoding region of protooncogene *fos* converts it to a transforming gene. *Proc. Natl. Acad. Sci. U.S.A.*, 82:4987–4991.
75. Miller, A.D., Curran, T., and Verma, I.M. (1984): c-*fos* Protein can induce cellular transformation: A novel mechanism of activation of a cellular oncogene. *Cell*, 36:51–60.
76. Miller, A.D., Verma, I.M., and Curran, T. (1985): Deletion of the *gag* region from FBR murine osteosarcoma virus does not affect its enhanced transforming activity. *J. Virol.*, 55:521–526.
77. Moscovici, C., Samarut, J., Gazzolo, L., and Moscovici, M.G. (1981): Myeloid and erythroid neoplastic responses to avian defective leukemia viruses in chickens and in quail. *Virology*, 113:765–768.
78. Naharro, G., Dunn, C.Y., and Robbins, K.C. (1983): Anaysis of the primary translational product and integrated DNA of a new feline sarcoma virus, GR-FeSV. *Virology*, 125:502–507.
79. Naharro, G., Robbins, K.C., and Reddy, E.P. (1984): Gene product of v-*fgr onc*: Hybrid protein containing a portion of actin and a tyrosine-specific protein kinase. *Science*, 223:63–66.
80. Naharro, G., Tronick, S.R., Rasheed, S., Gardner, M.B., Aaronson, S.A., and Robbins, K.C. (1983): Molecular cloning of integrated Gardner-Rasheed feline sarcoma virus: Genetic structure of its cell-derived sequence differs from that of other tyrosine kinase-coding *onc* genes. *J. Virol.*, 47:611–619.
81. Nilsen, T.W., Maroney, P.A., Goodwin, R.G., Rottman, F.M., Crittenden, L.B., Raines, M.A., and Kung, H.-J. (1985): c-*erb*B Activation in ALV-induced erythroblastosis: Novel RNA processing and promoter insertion result in expression of an amino-truncated EGF receptor. *Cell*, 41:719–726.
82. Nishida, T., Sakamoto, S., Yamamoto, T., Hayman, M., Kawai, S., and Toyoshima, K. (1984): Comparison of genome structures among three different strains of avian erythroblastosis virus. *Gann*, 75:325–333.
83. Nudel, U., Zakut, R., Shani, M., Neuman, S., Levy, Z., and Yaffe, D. (1983): The nucleotide sequence of the rat cytoplasmic β-actin gene. *Nucl. Acids Res.*, 11:1759–1771.
84. Nunn, M.F., Seeburg, P.H., Moscovici, C., and Duesberg, P.H. (1983): Tripartite structure of the avian erythroblastosis virus E26 transforming gene. *Nature*, 306:391–395.
85. Nunn, M., Weiher, H., Bullock, P., and Duesberg, P.H. (1984): Avian erythroblastosis virus E26: Nucleotide sequence of the tripartite *onc* gene and of the LTR, and analysis of the cellular prototype of the viral *ets* sequence. *Virology*, 139:330–339.
86. Pachl, C., Biegalke, B., and Linial, M. (1983): RNA and protein encoded by MH2 virus: Evidence for subgenomic expression of v-*myc*. *J. Virol.*, 45:133–139.
87. Palmieri, S., Beug, H., and Graf, T. (1982): Isolation and characterization of four new temperature-sensitive mutants of avian erythroblastosis virus (AEV). *Virology*, 123:296–311.
88. Parker, R.C., Varmus, H.E., and Bishop, J.M. (1984): Expression of v-*src* and chicken c-*src* in rat cells demonstrates qualitative differences between pp60$^{v\text{-}src}$ and pp60$^{c\text{-}src}$. *Cell*, 37:131–139.
89. Patschinsky, T., Jansen, H.W., Blöcker, H., Frank, R., and Bister, K. (1986): Structure and transforming function of transduced mutant alleles of the chicken c-*myc* gene. *J. Virol.*, 59:341–353.
90. Patschinsky, T., Schroeer, B., and Bister, K. (1986): Protein product of protooncogene c-*mil*. *Mol. Cell. Biol.*, 6:739–744.
91. Patschinsky, T., Walter, G., and Bister, K. (1984): Immunological analysis of v-*myc* gene products using antibodies against a *myc*-specific synthetic peptide. *Virology*, 136:348–358.
92. Privalsky, M.L., and Bishop, J.M. (1982): Proteins specified by avian erythroblastosis virus: Coding region localization and identification of a previously undetected *erb*-B polypeptide. *Proc. Natl. Acad. Sci. U.S.A.*, 79:3958–3962.
93. Radke, K., Beug, H., Kornfeld, S., and Graf, T. (1982): Transformation of both erythroid and myeloid cells by E26, an avian leukemia virus that contains the *myb* gene. *Cell*, 31:643–653.
94. Ramsay, G., Hayman, M.J., and Bister, K. (1982): Phosphorylation of specific sites in the *gag-myc* polyproteins encoded by MC29-type viruses correlates with their transforming ability. *EMBO J.*, 1:1111–1116.
95. Rapp, U.R., Cleveland, J.L., Brightman, K., Scott, A., and Ihle, J.N. (1985): Abrogation of IL-3 and IL-2 dependence by recombinant murine retroviruses expressing v-*myc* oncogenes. *Nature*, 317:434–438.

96. Rapp, U.R., Cleveland, J.L., Fredrickson, T.N., Holmes, K.L., Morse, III, H.C., Jansen, H.W., Patschinsky, T., and Bister, K. (1985): Rapid induction of hemopoietic neoplasms in newborn mice by a *raf(mil)/myc* recombinant murine retrovirus. *J. Virol.*, 55:23–33.

97. Rapp, U.R., Goldsborough, M.D., Mark, G.E., Bonner, T.I., Groffen, J., Reynolds, Jr., F.H., and Stephenson, J.R. (1983): Structure and biological activity of v-*raf*, a unique oncogene transduced by a retrovirus. *Proc. Natl. Acad. Sci. U.S.A.*, 80:4218–4222.

98. Rapp, U.R., Reynolds, Jr., F.H., and Stephenson, J.R. (1983): New mammalian transforming retrovirus: Demonstration of a polyprotein gene product. *J. Virol.*, 45:914–924.

99. Reddy, E.P., Reynolds, R.K., Watson, D.K., Schultz, R.A., Lautenberger, J., and Papas, T.S. (1983): Nucleotide sequence analysis of the proviral genome of avian myelocytomatosis virus (MC29). *Proc. Natl. Acad. Sci. U.S.A.*, 80:2500–2504.

100. Schatzman, R.C., Evan, G.I., Privalsky, M.L., and Bishop, J.M. (1986): Orientation of the v-*erb*-B gene product in the plasma membrane. *Mol. Cell. Biol.*, 6:1329–1333.

101. Schwartz, D.E., Tizard, R., and Gilbert, W. (1983): Nucleotide sequence of Rous sarcoma virus. *Cell*, 32:853–869.

102. Sealy, L., Moscovici, G., Moscovici, C., and Bishop, J.M. (1983): Site-specific mutagenesis of avian erythroblastosis virus: v-*erb*-A Is not required for transformation of fibroblasts. *Virology*, 130:179–194.

103. Sealy, L., Privalsky, M.L., Moscovici, G., Moscovici, C., and Bishop, J.M. (1983): Site-specific mutagenesis of avian erythroblastosis virus: *erb*-B Is required for oncogenecity. *Virology*, 130:155–178.

104. Shalloway, D., Coussens, P.M., and Yaciuk, P. (1984): Overexpression of the c-*src* protein does not induce transformation of NIH 3T3 cells. *Proc. Natl. Acad. Sci. U.S.A.*, 81:7071–7075.

105. Shimizu, K., Nakatsu, Y., Sekiguchi, M., Hokamura, K., Tanaka, K., Terada, M., and Sugimura, T. (1985): Molecular cloning of an activated human oncogene, homologous to v-*raf*, from primary stomach cancer. *Proc. Natl. Acad. Sci. U.S.A.*, 82:5641–5645.

106. Shtivelman, E., Lifshitz, B., Gale, R.P., and Canaani, E. (1985): Fused transcript of *abl* and *bcr* genes in chronic myelogenous leukaemia. *Nature*, 315:550–554.

107. Sotirov, N. (1981): Histone H5 in the immature blood cells of chickens with leukosis induced by avian leukosis virus strain E26. *J. Natl. Cancer Inst.*, 66:1143–1148.

108. Sutrave, P., Bonner, T.I., Rapp, U.R., Jansen, H.W., Patschinsky, T., and Bister, K. (1984): Nucleotide sequence of avian retroviral oncogene v-*mil*: Homologue of murine retroviral oncogene v-*raf*. *Nature*, 309:85–88.

109. Sutrave, P., Jansen, H.W., Bister, K., and Rapp, U.R. (1984): 3′-Terminal region of avian carcinoma virus MH2 shares sequence elements with avian sarcoma viruses Y73 and SR-A. *J. Virol.*, 52:703–705.

109a. Symonds, G., Quintrell, N., Stubblefield, E., and Bishop, J.M. (1986): Dispersed chromosomal localization of the proto-oncogenes transduced into the genome of Mill Hill 2 or E26 leukemia virus. *J. Virol.*, 59:172–175.

110. Symonds, G., Stubblefield, E., Guyaux, M., and Bishop, J.M. (1984): Cellular oncogenes (c-*erb*-A and c-*erb*-B) located on different chicken chromosomes can be transduced into the same retroviral genome. *Mol. Cell. Biol.*, 4:1627–1630.

111. Takeya, T., and Hanafusa, H. (1983): Structure and sequence of the cellular gene homologous to the RSV *src* gene and the mechanism for generating the transforming virus. *Cell*, 32:881–890.

112. Temin, H.M. (1984): Do we understand the genetic mechanisms of oncogenesis? *J. Cell. Physiol. [Suppl.]*, 3:1–11.

113. Tronick, S.R., Popescu, N.C., Cheah, M.S.C., Swan, D.C., Amsbaugh, S.C., Lengel, C.R., DiPaolo, J.A., and Robbins, K.C. (1985): Isolation and chromosomal localization of the human *fgr* protooncogene, a distinct member of the tyrosine kinase gene family. *Proc. Natl. Acad. Sci. U.S.A.*, 82:6595–6599.

114. Ullrich, A., Coussens, L., Hayflick, J.S., Dull, T.J., Gray, A., Tam, A.W., Lee, J., Yarden, Y., Libermann, T.A., Schlessinger, J., Downward, J., Mayes, E.L.V., Whittle, N., Waterfield, M.D., and Seeburg, P.H. (1984): Human epidermal growth factor receptor cDNA sequence and aberrant expression of the amplified gene in A431 epidermoid carcinoma cells. *Nature*, 309:418–425.

115. Van Beveren, C., Enami, S., Curran, T., and Verma, I.M. (1984): FBR murine osteosarcoma virus. II. Nucleotide sequence of the provirus reveals that the genome contains sequences acquired from two cellular genes. *Virology*, 135:229–243.

116. Van Beveren, C., Van Straaten, F., Curran, T., Müller, R., and Verma, I.M. (1983): Analysis

of FBJ-MuSV provirus and *c-fos* (mouse) gene reveals that viral and cellular *fos* gene products have different carboxy termini. *Cell,* 32:1241–1255.

117. Vandekerckhove, J., and Weber, K. (1978): Mammalian cytoplasmic actins are the products of at least two genes and differ in primary structure in at least 25 identified positions from skeletal muscle actins. *Proc. Natl. Acad. Sci. U.S.A.,* 75:1106–1110.

118. Varmus, H.E. (1984): The molecular genetics of cellular oncogenes. *Annu. Rev. Genet.,* 18:553–612.

119. Vennström, B., Fanshier, L., Moscovici, C., and Bishop, J.M. (1980): Molecular cloning of the avian erythroblastosis virus genome and recovery of oncogenic virus by transfection of chicken cells. *J. Virol.,* 36:575–585.

120. Vogt, P.K. (1977): Genetics of RNA tumor viruses. In: *Comprehensive Virology, Vol. 9,* edited by H. Fraenkel-Conrat and R.R. Wagner, pp. 341–455. Plenum Press, New York.

121. Walther, N., Lurz, R., Patschinsky, T., Jansen, H.W., and Bister, K. (1985): Molecular cloning of proviral DNA and structural analysis of the transduced *myc* oncogene of avian oncovirus CMII. *J. Virol.,* 54:576–585.

122. Walther, N., Jansen, H.W., Trachmann, C., and Bister, K. (1986): Nucleotide sequence of the CMII v-*myc* allele. *Virology,* 159:219–223.

122a. Watson, D.K., McWilliams-Smith, M.J., Nunn, M.F., Duesberg, P.H., O'Brien, S.J., and Papas, T.S. (1985): The *ets* sequence from the transforming gene of avian erythroblastosis virus, E26, has unique domains on human chromosomes 11 and 21: Both loci are transcriptionally active. *Proc. Natl. Acad. Sci. U.S.A.,* 82:7294–7298.

123. Watson, D.K., Reddy, E.P., Duesberg, P.H., and Papas, T.S. (1983): Nucleotide sequence analysis of the chicken c-*myc* gene reveals homologous and unique coding regions by comparison with the transforming gene of avian myelocytomatosis virus MC29, Δ*gag-myc*. *Proc. Natl. Acad. Sci. U.S.A.,* 80:2146–2150.

124. Weinberger, C., Hollenberg, S.M., Rosenfeld, M.G., and Evans, R.M. (1985): Domain structure of human glucocorticoid receptor and its relationship to the v-*erb*-A oncogene product. *Nature,* 318:670–672.

124a. Yaciuk, P., and Shalloway, D. (1986): Features of the pp60$^{v\text{-}src}$ carboxyl terminus that are required for transformation. *Mol. Cell. Biol.,* 6:2807–2819.

125. Yamamoto, T., Hihara, H., Nishida, T., Kawai, S., and Toyoshima, K. (1983): A new avian erythroblastosis virus, AEV-H, carries *erbB* gene responsible for the induction of both erythroblastosis and sarcomas. *Cell,* 34:225–232.

126. Zhou, R.-P., Kan, N., Papas, T., and Duesberg, P. (1985): Mutagenesis of avian carcinoma virus MH2: Only one of two potential transforming genes (δ*gag-myc*) transforms fibroblasts. *Proc. Natl. Acad. Sci. U.S.A.,* 82:6389–6393.

Advances in Viral Oncology, Volume 6, edited by
George Klein, Raven Press, New York © 1987.

Sequences that Influence the Transforming Activity and Expression of the *mos* Oncogene

George F. Vande Woude, Marianne Oskarsson, Mary Lou McGeady, Arun Seth, Friedrich Propst, Martin Schmidt, Richard Paules, and Donald G. Blair

Litton Bionetics, Inc.-Basic Research Program, National Cancer Institute-Frederick Cancer Research Facility, Frederick, Maryland 21701

The viral and cellular homologs of the *mos* oncogene have been useful for studying the molecular elements required for cell transformation. These studies provided the first direct comparison of a viral oncogene and its cellular counterpart (14,20) and demonstrated that the cellular *mos* could be activated by viral sequences to cause cell transformation (20). It was subsequently shown that the proviral transcription element or long terminal repeat (LTR), specifically the LTR enhancer sequence, was responsible for activation of the transforming potential of the mouse *mos* oncogene (c-*mos*^mu) (2,3,17,32). The more difficult problem of identifying the mechanisms by which the *mos* oncogene causes expression of the transformed phenotype remains to be solved. One approach to this problem has been to study proto-oncogene expression, which can reveal important information about oncogene function. The discovery that the *fms* oncogene is the CSF-1 receptor (24) is one example of a correlation that was made based on proto-oncogene expression. Previously, however, the lack of evidence for *mos* proto-oncogene expression in normal tissues had prevented the use of this approach (9,11,19) [only recently have c-*mos* transcripts been detected in normal tissues (22)]. Prior to this observation we studied the biological transforming activity of the LTR-activated c-*mos* as a means of identifying transcription regulatory elements within the normal locus. Indeed, the first indication of such a regulatory element was observed in the early attempts to activate the c-*mos*^mu with LTR elements placed either upstream or downstream of the oncogene. In these studies, constructs in which an LTR was placed downstream of *mos* were 1,000-fold lower in transforming activity than those in which *mos* was activated with an upstream LTR (20,31). An element called the upstream mouse sequence (UMS) located approximately 1,500 base pairs (bp) upstream to c-*mos*^mu, was subsequently shown to be responsible for inhibiting transforming activity. UMS appears to prevent transcription readthrough by acting as a transcription terminator (18a,31).

In this chapter, we describe regulatory sequences that can influence c-*mos* gene expression as detected by biological transformation assays. The c-*mos*^mu sequences have been most extensively characterized, but we shall also describe how assays comparing the transforming activities of c-*mos* genes isolated from the mouse, human (c-*mos*[hu]), and chicken (c-*mos*[ch]) genomes have been useful for identifying regulatory sequences as well as for identifying important functional domains in the *mos* protein.

The conservation of the *mos* open reading frame strongly suggests that the gene must function during the life cycle (26,27,29). This observation, coupled with the low level of *mos* RNA expression observed both in some v-*mos*-transformed cells (30,32) and in plasmacytoma tumor cell lines with *mos* activated by insertional mutagenesis (7,10,23) together with the putative toxic effects of high levels of *mos* protein expression (21), suggest that the *mos* proto-oncogene may be expressed in normal tissues at very low levels. These properties also indicate that *mos* is one of the most potent of the transforming genes, one reason why we have maintained a keen interest in studying the gene. Studying *mos* presents special difficulties, however, because the low levels of *mos* expression often test the limits of our most sensitive assays.

UPSTREAM MOUSE SEQUENCE: A TRANSCRIPTION REGULATOR

We have shown that activation of c-*mos*[mu] by a downstream LTR is prevented by the normal mouse sequences (UMS) preceding the oncogene (31). This inhibitory sequence, an AT-rich region less than 600 bp long, is located more than 1,500 bp upstream of the conserved c-*mos*[mu] ATG initiation codon. We also demonstrated that the UMS could prevent activation of v-*mos* by a downstream LTR only when it was inserted between viral sequences, which serve as a promoter, and the ATG of the viral oncogene. The results of these studies are summarized in Fig. 1. The UMS appears to prevent transcripts from transcribing into *mos* when there is no transcriptional promoter between UMS and *mos*. This observation proved to be valuable, for it allowed us to identify the region responsible for promoting v-*mos* transcripts (31). In a few NIH/3T3 cell transformants transformed with v-*mos* and a downstream LTR, Wood *et al.* (32) observed low expression of v-*mos*, estimated to be one to 10 transcripts per cell; however, most transformants expressed abundant and complex v-*mos* transcription patterns. Transformants exhibiting the aberrant transcripts had acquired efficient upstream promoters during transfection from either host or carrier DNA sequences. It was reasoned that these transcripts were either inefficiently translated or prevented detection of the true functional *mos* transcript. Evidence supporting this model was obtained by placing UMS upstream to a region where viral sequences could serve as a promoter for v-*mos*. The only transcripts observed in transformants obtained by transfecting this construct originated from viral sequences that could act as a promoter, and these were expressed at low levels (31).

These studies also indicated that there is no promoter that functions in the NIH/3T3 cells used for the transformation assay in the 2-kilobase (kb) span of nucleotide sequences upstream of the c-*mos*[mu] proto-oncogene. This finding sug-

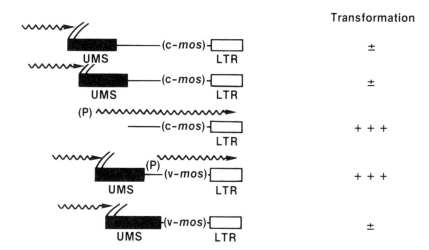

FIG. 1. The influence of UMS on c-mos^mu and v-mos expression. The difference of ± to + + + represents a 50- to 100-fold increase in transforming activity: (P) *mos* promoter; *(wavy arrows)* transcript. The drawing summarizes results as presented in Wood *et al.* (31).

gested among other possibilities that the c-*mos*^mu proto-oncogene transcription unit might be activated in *trans* (31). Further characterization of the UMS (18a) shows that it possesses two functional polyadenylation sites and that when UMS is placed downstream from a transcription locus, it has activity analogous to that proposed for transcription termination signals (6). Thus, UMS may be a transcription terminator for some upstream, still unidentified, gene locus. It is also possible that UMS functions merely to restrict transcription into the c-*mos*^mu locus in certain cell types, since low-level expression of *mos* in cells such as NIH/3T3 cells can result in the expression of its transforming potential. In these cases, UMS would function in *cis* as a negative regulatory element. However, transcripts containing UMS may be expressed in certain tissues (22), and under these circumstances UMS may be positively regulated to either allow expression of the *mos* proto-oncogene or, at least, not interfere with *mos* expression. Although UMS is not conserved in the c-*mos*^hu locus, homology to UMS has been reported in other species (28), suggesting that the regulation of *mos* proto-oncogene transcription in these other species may be similar to c-*mos*^mu.

c-*mos*^hu ACTIVATION AND REGULATORY SEQUENCES

Early attempts to activate the transforming potential of c-*mos*^hu with LTR sequences were unsuccessful, even though the amino acid sequence of human proto-oncogene was 75% conserved (29). The human homolog possesses an overlapping open reading frame (29) that precedes the *mos* ATG. Transfection assays of recombinant DNA constructs containing hybrid human/mouse *mos* genes (4) demonstrated that removal of sequences immediately upstream of the human ATG could enhance the transforming activity by several orders of magnitude (2a). We therefore tested c-*mos*[hu] activation with an LTR element placed within 25 bp of the conserved *mos* ATG, thereby eliminating the overlapping open reading frame (Fig. 2) (2a). These constructs, pLh 4, 22, 23, 24, and pLhT, which eliminated all but approximately 25 bases between the LTR and the c-*mos*[hu] open reading frame, all exhibited transforming activity. However, the most active c-*mos*[hu] recombinants were 20- to 50-fold lower than similar c-*mos*[mu] constructs, and the foci were distinguishable from v-*mos* foci in that they were smaller and contained fewer cells with refractile morphology (Table 1) (2a). When the LTR was positioned farther upstream of the c-*mos*[hu] ATG, as in pPHT (250 bp) (Fig. 2), the activity decreased more than 15-fold. One interpretation of these data is that eliminating the overlapping open reading frame allows more efficient expression of c-*mos*[hu] protein, which is less efficient as a transforming protein (2a,4). It is also possible that UMS-like sequences are present in this region.

IDENTIFICATION OF ACTIVITY DOMAINS IN HYBRID c-*mos*[mu]/c-*mos*[hu] GENES

The marked differences in the transforming efficiencies of c-*mos*[hu] and c-*mos*[mu] have been attributed to differences in the protein coding region (2a,4). We have constructed hybrid human and mouse *mos* genes in an attempt to identify the domains responsible for these differences. By analyzing the transforming activity of hybrid *mos* gene constructs, we obtained evidence for three domains in the *mos*

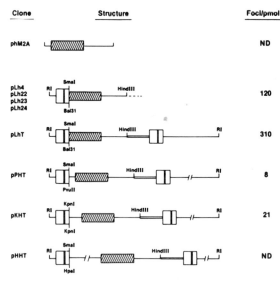

FIG. 2. Structure and biological activity of constructs containing human c-*mos*. The activity is based on the average of at least four separate transfections. The structural features of the constructs containing *mos* are as shown: *(hatched areas)* human sequences homologous to *mos*; *(open areas)* murine sarcoma virus LTR-derived sequences; R1 = *Eco*RI. The relative positions of restriction sites are indicated.

TABLE 1. mos *Transforming efficiencies*[a]

Plasmid	mos Species	Structure[c]	Focus-forming units per picomote
pLh04	c-mos[hu]	□–( )	54
pTS1[b]	c-mos[mu]	□—( )	2,572
pM1CM33	c-mos[ch]	□–( )	1,166
pM1CM36	c-mos[ch]	□——( )	239

[a]Data from ref. 25.
[b]Data from ref. 3.
[c](□) Position of LTR sequences relative to the designated mos ( ) gene.

coding region that can influence transforming efficiency. The results from these analyses can be summarized by comparing amino acid sequences of c-*mos*[hu] and c-*mos*[mu] (Fig. 3). The first domain from c-*mos*[mu] that can increase transforming efficiency in hybrid *mos* genes is situated between positions 48 and 80 (all positions in Fig. 3 correspond to numbering of c-*mos*[hu] codons). In this stretch of 32 amino acids, there are only five amino acid differences between the two *mos* genes. It is interesting that three of the five amino acid differences (at positions 68, 73, 80) cluster in a region where there is extensive homology among *mos*, *src,* and bovine cyclic AMP-dependent protein kinase (1) (position 66–74). This consensus region is just upstream from a conserved lysine at position 87, which is the proposed ATP-binding site for the bovine kinase and *mos* (12). The *mos* protein produced in *Escherichia coli* has been shown to bind ATP (25), and it is possible that differences in the amino acids of the human and mouse domains affect ATP binding and hence influence transforming activity.

The second domain has been localized between positions 155 and 172, a region of total nonhomology in the two species. It has been observed that when the amino acid sequence C-terminal to this domain is not from the homologous species, there is a marked decrease in biological activity, suggesting that the domain must interact in some fashion with the C-terminal portion of the molecule (2a,4). That this nonconserved region should be functionally important for transforming activity was unexpected.

Although these two domains can influence the transforming activity of hybrid *mos* genes, a third domain representing the C-terminal moiety of the protein (i.e., from position 223–346) appears to have the most significant effect. There are numerous amino acid differences in this domain, but this is the region that possesses homology with the *src* kinase domain (13). The significant influence of the C-terminal moiety on transforming activity, its relatedness to the *src* kinase domain, plus evidence indicating that the *mos* product is a serine kinase (16,18) suggest that the third domain is an important functional domain of the protein.

FIG. 3. Comparison of the deduced amino acid sequences of c-mos[hu], c-mos[mu] and c-mos[ch]. Each domain, 1–111, is defined by arrows and based on data from Blair et al. (2a,4). The sequences are from Van Beveren et al. (26) for c-mos[mu], Watson et al. (29) for c-mos[hu] and M. Schmidt (unpublished data, 1986) for c-mos[ch].

```
c-mos^hu   1    M P S P L A L R P Y L R S E F S P S V D A R P C S S P S E L P       A K L L L G
c-mos^mu   1    M P S P L S L C R Y L P R E L S P S V D S R C S S I P L V A P P R K A G K L F L G
c-mos^ch   1    M P S P I P F N S F L P L E F S P S A D L R P C S S P V V I P G K D G K A F L G

                                                DOMAIN 1

c-mos^hu   38   A T L P R A P R L   P R R L A W C S I D W E Q V C L L Q R L G A G G F G S V Y K
c-mos^mu   41   T T P P R A P G L   P R R L A W F S I D W E Q V C L M H R L G S G G F G S V Y K
c-mos^ch   41   G T P S P R T R R L P P R L A W C S I D W D R L C L L Q P L G S G G F G A V Y K

c-mos^hu   77   A T Y R G V P V A I K Q V N K C T K N R L A S R R S F W A E L N V A R L R H D N
c-mos^mu   80   A T Y H G V P V A I K Q V N K C T K D L R A S Q R S F W A E L N I A R L R H D N
c-mos^ch   81   A T Y H G V T V A V K Q V K Q V K S S K N R L A S R Q S F W A E L N V A R L Q H D N

c-mos^hu   117  I V R V V A A S T R T P A G S N S L G T I I M E F G G N V T L H Q V I Y G A A G
c-mos^mu   120  I V R V V A A S T R T P E D S N S L G T I I M E F G G N V T L H Q V I Y G A T R
c-mos^ch   121  V V R V V A A S T C A P A S Q N S L G T I I M E Y V G N V T L H H V I Y G   T R

                                                DOMAIN 2

c-mos^hu   157  H P E G D A G E P H C R T G G Q L S L G K C L K Y S L D V V N G L L F L H S Q
c-mos^mu   160  S P E   P L S C   R E Q L S L G K C L K Y S L D V V N G L L F L H S Q
c-mos^ch   160  D A W R Q G E E E G G C G R K A L S M A E A V C Y S C D I V T G L A F L H S Q

c-mos^hu   196  S I V H L D L K P A N I L I S E Q D V C K I S D F G C S E K L E D L L C F Q T P
c-mos^mu   193  S I L H L D L K P A N I L I S E Q D V C K I S D F G C S Q K L Q V L R C R Q A S
c-mos^ch   200  G I V H L D L K P A N I L I T E H G A C K I G D F G C S Q R L E E G L S Q S H H

                                                DOMAIN 3

c-mos^hu   236  S Y P L G G T Y T H R A P E L L K G E V T P K A D I Y S F A I T L W Q M T T K
c-mos^mu   233  P H H I G G T Y T H Q A P E L L K G E I A T P K A D I Y S F G I T L W Q M T T R
c-mos^ch   240  V C Q Q G G T Y T H R A P E L L K G E R V T A K A D I Y S F A I T L W Q I V M R

c-mos^hu   276  Q A P Y S G E R Q H I L Y A V V A Y D L R P S L S A A V F E D S L P G Q R L G D
c-mos^mu   273  E V P Y S G E P Q Y V V Q V A V V A Y N L R P S L A G A V F T A S L T G K T L Q N
c-mos^ch   280  E Q P Y L G E R Q Y V L Y A V A Y N L R P P L A A A I F H E S A V G Q R L R S

c-mos^hu   316  V I I Q R C W R P S A A Q R P S A R L L L V D L T S L K A E L G       346
c-mos^mu   313  I I Q S C W E A R A L Q R P G A E L L Q R D L K A F R G A L G       343
c-mos^ch   320  I I S C C W K A D V E E R L S A A Q L L P S L R A L K E N L       349
```

c-*mos*[ch] AMINO ACID SEQUENCE COMPARISON AND ACTIVATION

The transforming activity of LTR-activated c-*mos*[hu] is relatively low in comparison to c-*mos*[mu]; however, the c-*mos*[ch] has almost the same transforming activity as LTR-activated c-*mos*[mu] (pM1CM33; Table 1) (M. Schmidt, *unpublished data,* 1986). These data also show that when the LTR is placed 900 bp upstream of c-*mos*[ch] (pM1CM36), the transforming activity is five- to tenfold lower than when in close proximity (pM1CM33) and suggests that the presence of a negative regulatory sequence is also upstream of c-*mos*[ch]. However, nucleotide sequence analysis of this locus shows no homology to either the human or mouse upstream sequences other than the fact that they are all AT rich (M. Schmidt, *unpublished data,* 1986).

The higher activity of c-*mos*[ch] than of c-*mos*[hu] is surprising, since c-*mos*[ch] is less homologous to c-*mos*[mu] (62%) than is c-*mos*[hu] (75%) (Fig. 3). Moreover, compared to other oncogenes that have been studied, *mos* is unusual in that it has far less amino acid sequence homology conserved between species. Perhaps the extensive changes that have occurred indicate that the targets of the *mos* product are not tightly conserved as could be implied from the extensive conservation of, for example, the *ras* family of oncogenes (8,15). Since parallel divergence of a protein with its target is improbable, this suggests that the transforming activity of *mos* protein is due to an intrinsic property and that its target(s) is a small molecule or it has a larger target that diverges more rapidly than proteins (i.e., nucleic acid sequences).

There are only 184 codons in c-*mos*[ch] that are conserved in the other two species; however, 50 additional codons are conserved in c-*mos*[mu] or c-*mos*[hu] (22 and 28, respectively). If the transforming efficiencies of the three different *mos* genes can be equated with the differences in amino acid sequence in the three domains described (Fig. 3), then the identification of specific amino acid differences may serve to pinpoint active sites. For example, in the first, or ATP-binding, domain, the only significant difference between c-*mos*[hu] and the efficiently transforming c-*mos*[mu] and c-*mos*[ch] is at position 68. This is in the consensus sequence (LGX-GXFGXV) for the ATP-binding site (1), where alanine is present in the c-*mos*[hu] sequence, and serine is present in the others. The other four differences in the c-*mos*[hu] (cf. c-*mos*[mu]) sequence are either conservative changes or, by virtue of their homology with the c-*mos*[ch] sequence, may not influence or contribute to the transforming activity of the protein. Similar deductions can be made in the third domain, but obviously all of these interpretations must be viewed circumspectly until appropriate site-directed mutagenesis studies are performed.

Finally, the relative inefficiency of c-*mos*[hu] as a transforming gene may be significant, since conceivably it could provide the species with a selective advantage. If *mos* transforming activity reflects its activity as a proto-oncogene; however, we would then expect its function in humans to be less active. One way to overcome this problem would be to have other protein(s) evolve that can augment its activity; however, the possibility that c-*mos*[hu] is an efficient transforming gene in specific human cells has not been explored.

c-*mos*[mu] EXPRESSION

The discovery of c-*mos* proto-oncogene transcripts in normal tissues (22) should lead to a better understanding of its normal function; however, the transcription pattern, as depicted in Fig. 4, is unique and clearly complex. First, the level of expression in all tissues is very low, ranging from approximately 10 copies per cell to less than one copy per 10 cells (22; *unpublished data*). Moreover, the size of the transcript varies in a tissue-specific fashion, ranging from approximately 1.3 to 6 kb. All transcripts are 3' coterminal, and the variation in size is caused by differences at the 5' end (22; F. Propst, *unpublished data, 1986*). This suggests that different promoters are used in different tissues for *mos* expression. Thus far, there is no evidence for RNA processing of intervening sequences (F. Propst, *unpublished data, 1986*), which leaves the c-*mos* open reading frame in most tissues as the only coding exon. We do not know if additional coding regions other than *mos* exist, for example, in the 6-kb transcript. Each transcript in testes and ovaries contains only the *mos* open reading frame and cannot give rise to products larger than the *mos* product that causes transformation of NIH/3T3 cells. Obviously, in gonadal tissue its transforming activity is suppressed, and other mechanisms must be responsible for its transforming activity in other tissues. Perhaps, then, the mere expression of *mos* in the wrong cells or tissue types may cause expression of its transforming potential.

Curiously, the 1.3-kb class of transcripts detected in whole-mouse-embryo RNA appears to start within the *mos* coding region, and a protein expressed from such transcripts would have to initiate at methionine at position 64 (Fig. 3) in c-*mos*[mu]. It has been demonstrated, however, that initiation at methionine still yields a transforming gene product (5).

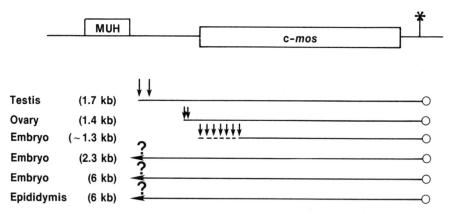

FIG. 4. *mos* Proto-oncogene transcripts in mouse tissues. The transcript size determinations and properties are described in Propst and Vande Woude (22). MUH is a conserved nucleotide sequence upstream of the c-*mos*[mu] and c-*mos*[mu] open reading frames (4). The *arrows* indicate putative start sites; *asterisk* approximates the position downstream of *mos* containing a consensus polyadenylation site and signal (26).

A region upstream to *mos*, termed mouse upstream homology (MUH) (4), is 75% homologous in nucleic acid sequences in c-*mos*^{mu} and c-*mos*^{hu}. We believe that c-*mos*^{mu} testes transcripts initiate just downstream from this conserved region (22; F. Probst, *unpublished data*, 1986), and MUH (4), as previously speculated, may play a role in regulating expression. It is very likely that the larger transcript (6 kb) contains sequences transcribed from UMS (22). This transcript has not been extensively characterized, and it is not known whether UMS sequences are present or are processed as an intron, but neither polyadenylation nor transcription termination could function in UMS in these tissues.

Collectively, these analyses show that *mos* gene transcription is regulated in a very novel fashion. There are few or no examples of the mechanisms that regulate the expression of genes transcribed at the level of a few copies per cell, although it may not be uncommon for genes expressed at this level to be regulated in such a fashion. However, the other properties we have described for the *mos* gene are equally unusual. There are few conserved genes in eukaryotic cells that lack intervening sequences, and, as mentioned above, the *mos* product is both very efficient as a transforming protein and is perhaps, compared to other oncogene proteins, novel in the way that it transforms cells. This fact, coupled with its low expression in normal tissues, makes it more likely that *mos* has evolved in a very distinct manner with regard to regulatory sequences.

ACKNOWLEDGMENTS

Research was sponsored by the National Cancer Institute, Department of Health and Human Services, under Contract No. N01-CO-23909 with Litton Bionetics, Inc. The contents of this publication do not necessarily reflect the views or policies of the Department of Health and Human Services, nor does mention of trade names, commercial products, or organizations imply endorsement by the U.S. Government.

REFERENCES

1. Barker, W.C., and Dayhoff, M.O. (1982): Viral *src* gene products are related to the catalytic chain of mammalian cAMP-dependent protein kinase. *Proc. Natl. Acad. Sci. U.S.A.,* 79:2836–2839.
2. Blair, D.G., McClements, W.L., Oskarsson, M.K., Fischinger, P.J., and Vande Woude, G.F. (1980): Biological activity of cloned Moloney sarcoma virus DNA: Terminally redundant sequences may enhance transformation efficiency. *Proc. Natl. Acad. Sci. U.S.A.,* 77:3504–3508.
2a. Blair, D.G., Oskarsson, M.K., Seth, A., Dunn, K.J., Dean, M., Zweig, M., and Vande Woude, G.F. (1986): Analysis of the transforming potential of the human homolog of *mos.* *(in press).*
3. Blair, D.G., Oskarsson, M., Wood, T.G., McClements, W.L., Fischinger, P.J., and Vande Woude, G.F. (1981): Activation of the transforming potential of a normal cell sequence: A molecular model for oncogenesis. *Science,* 212:941–943.
4. Blair, D.G., Wood, T.G., Woodworth, A.M., McGeady, M.L., Oskarsson, M.K., Propst, F., Tainsky, M., Cooper, C.S., Watson, R., Baroudy, B.M., and Vande Woude, G.F. (1984): Properties of the mouse and human *mos* oncogene loci. In: *Cancer Cells: Oncogenes and Viral Genes,*

Vol. 2, edited by G.F. Vande Woude, A.J. Levine, W.C. Topp, and J.D. Watson, pp. 281–289. Cold Spring Harbor Laboratory, Cold Spring Harbor, New York.

5. Bold, R.J., and Donoghue, D.J. (1985): Biologically active mutants with deletions in the v-*mos* oncogene assayed with retroviral vectors. *Mol. Cell. Biol.,* 5:3131–3138.

6. Citron, B., Flack-Pederson, E., Salditt-Georgieff, M., and Darnell, Jr., J.E. (1984): Transcription termination occurs within a 1,000-base-pair region downstream from the poly(A) site of the mouse B-globin (major) gene. *Nucleic Acids Res.,* 12:8723–8731.

7. Cohen, J.B., Unger, T., Rechavi, G., Canaani, E., and Givol, D. (1983): Rearrangement of the oncogene c-*mos* in mouse myeloma NSI and hybridomas. *Nature,* 306:797–799.

8. DeFeo-Jones, D., Tatchell, K., Robinson, L.C., Sigal, I.S., Vass, W.C., Lowy, D.R., and Scolnick, E.M. (1985): Mammalian and yeast *ras* gene products: Biological function in their heterologous systems. *Science,* 228:179–184.

9. Gattoni, S., Kirschmeier, P., Weinstein, I.B., Escobedo, J., and Dina, D. (1982): Cellular Moloney murine sarcoma (c-*mos*) sequences are hypermethylated and transcriptionally silent in normal and transformed rodent cells. *Mol. Cell. Biol.,* 2:45–51.

10. Gattoni-Celli, S., Hsiao, W.-L.W., and Weinstein, I.B. (1983): Rearranged c-*mos* locus in a MOPC 21 murine myeloma cell line and its persistence in hybridomas. *Nature,* 306:795–796.

11. Goyette, M., Petropoulos, C.J., Shank, P.R., and Fausto, N. (1984): Regulated transcription of c-Ki-*ras* and c-*myc* during compensatory growth of rat liver. *Mol. Cell. Biol.,* 4:1493–1498.

12. Hannik, M., and Donoghue, D.J. (1985): Lysine residue 121 in the proposed ATP-binding site of the v-*mos* protein is required for transformation. *Proc. Natl. Acad. Sci. U.S.A.,* 82:7894–7898.

13. Hunter, T., and Cooper, J.A. (1986): Viral oncogenes and tyrosine phosphorylation. In: *The Enzymes; Enzyme Control by Protein Phosphorylation,* edited by P.D. Boyer and E.G. Krebs. Academic Press, New York. *(In press.)*

14. Jones, M., Bosselman, R.A., van der Hoorn, F.A., Berns, A., Fan, H., and Verma, I.M. (1980): Identification and molecular cloning of Moloney mouse sarcoma virus-specific sequences from uninfected mouse cells. *Proc. Natl. Acad. Sci. U.S.A.,* 77:2651–2655.

15. Kataoka, T., Powers, S., Cameron, S., Fasano, O., Goldfarb, M., Broach, J., and Wigler, M. (1985): Functional homology of mammalian and yeast *ras* genes. *Cell,* 40:19–26.

16. Kloetzer, W.S., Maxwell, S.A., and Arlinghaus, R.B. (1983): p85^gag-mos encoded by *ts*110 Moloney murine sarcoma virus has an associated protein kinase activity. *Proc. Natl. Acad. Sci. U.S.A.,* 80:412–416.

17. Levinson, B., Khoury, G., Vande Woude, G., and Gruss, P. (1982): Activation of the SV40 genome by the 72-base-pair tandem repeats of Moloney sarcoma virus. *Nature (London),* 295:568–572.

18. Maxwell, S.A., and Arlinghaus, R.B. (1985): Serine kinase activity associated with Moloney murine sarcoma virus-124-encoded p37^mos. *Virology,* 143:321–333.

18a. McGeady, M.L., Wood, T.C., Maizel, J.V., and Vande Woude, G.F. (1986): Sequences upstream to the mouse c-*mos* may function as a transcription signal. *DNA (in press.)*

19. Muller, R., Slamon, D.J., Tremblay, J.M., Cline, M.J., and Verma, I.M. (1982): Differential expression of cellular oncogenes during pre- and postnatal development of the mouse. *Nature,* 299:640–644.

20. Oskarsson, M., McClements, W.L., Blair, D.G., Maizel, J.V., and Vande Woude, G.F. (1980): Properties of a normal mouse cell DNA sequence (sarc) homologous to the src sequence of Moloney sarcoma virus. *Science,* 207:1222–1224.

21. Papkoff, J., Verma, I.M., and Hunter, T. (1982): Detection of a transforming gene product in cells transformed by Moloney murine sarcoma virus. *Cell,* 29:417–426.

22. Propst, F., and Vande Woude, G.F. (1985): Expression of c-*mos* proto-oncogene transcripts in mouse tissues. *Nature,* 315:516–518.

23. Rechavi, G., Givol, D., and Canaani, E. (1982): Activation of a cellular oncogene by DNA rearrangement. Possible involvement of an IS-like element. *Nature,* 300:607–611.

24. Scherr, C.J., Rettenmier, C.W., Sacca, R., Roussel, M.F., Look, A.T., and Stanley, E. (1985): The c-*fms* proto-oncogene product is related to the receptor for the mononuclear phagocyte growth factor, CSF-1. *Cell,* 41:665–676.

25. Seth, A., and Vande Woude, G.F. (1985): Nucleotide sequence and the biochemical activities of the HT1MSV *mos* gene. *J. Virol.,* 56:144–152.

26. Van Beveren, C., van Straaten, F., Galleshaw, J.A., and Verma, I.M. (1981): Nucleotide sequence of the genome of a murine sarcoma virus. *Cell,* 27:97–108.

27. Van der Hoorn, F.A., and Firzlaff, J. (1984): Complete c-*mos* rat nucleotide sequence: Presence of conserved domains in c-*mos* proteins. *Nucleic Acids Res.,* 12:2147–2156.

28. Van der Hoorn, F.A., Muller, V., and Pizer, L. (1985): Sequences upstream of c-*mos* (rat) that block RNA accumulation in mouse cells do not inhibit in vitro transcription. *Mol. Cell. Biol.,* 5:406–409.

29. Watson, R., Oskarsson, M., and Vande Woude, G.F. (1982): Human DNA sequence homologous to the transforming gene (*mos*) of Moloney murine sarcoma virus. *Proc. Natl. Acad. Sci. U.S.A.,* 79:4078–4082.

30. Wood, T.G., Blair, D.G., and Vande Woude, G.F. (1983): Moloney sarcoma virus: analysis of RNA and DNA structure in cells transformed by subgenomic proviral DNA fragments. In: *Perspectives on Genes and the Molecular Biology of Cancer,* edited by D.L. Robberson and G.F. Saunders, pp. 299–306. Raven Press, New York.

31. Wood, T.G., McGeady, M.L., Baroudy, B.M., Blair, D.G., and Vande Woude, G.F. (1984): Mouse c-*mos* oncogene activation is prevented by upstream sequences. *Proc. Natl. Acad. Sci. U.S.A.,* 81:7817–7821.

32. Wood, T.G., McGeady, M.L., Blair, D.G., and Vande Woude, G.F. (1983): Long terminal repeat enhancement of v-*mos* transforming activity: Identification of essential regions. *J. Virol.,* 46:726–736.

Advances in Viral Oncology,Volume 6, edited by
George Klein, Raven Press, New York © 1987.

Genetic Regulation of Tumorigenic Expression in Somatic Cell Hybrids

Eric J. Stanbridge

Department of Microbiology and Molecular Genetics, College of Medicine, University of California at Irvine, Irvine, California 92717

The technique of somatic cell hybridization, whereby somatic cell hybrids are generated by fusing together two or more different cells of the same or different species, was first applied to the study of the genetic analysis of malignancy more than 20 years ago. Intraspecies rodent, interspecies human-rodent, and intraspecies human cell hybrids have been used. In these studies, the general approach has been to fuse a cancer cell with a normal cell and determine whether or not the resulting hybrid is tumorigenic. The answer to this seemingly simple question has been the subject of considerable controversy. The major reason for this controversy has been the chromosomal instability of the aforementioned hybrid cells—a controversy that was laid to rest when it was shown that there is stable suppression of the malignant phenotype in intraspecies human cell hybrids. These human hybrid cells show remarkable chromosome stability. There have been several reviews of the earlier studies with somatic cell hybrids (27,42,63). I shall therefore focus on those studies of the past few years that have enlightened our understanding of the genetic control of malignancy in somatic cell hybrids. In order to acquaint the reader with some of the controversy that has swirled around the use of somatic cell hybrids, however, I shall begin with a brief historical overview of these somatic hybrid cell studies.

HISTORICAL ASPECTS OF SOMATIC CELL HYBRIDIZATION STUDIES

Early investigators in this field isolated hybrid cells derived from the fusion of mouse cells of low malignant potential with those of high malignant potential. The intraspecific mouse cell hybrids derived from these fusions were as malignant as the highly malignant parent, thereby leading to the interpretation that malignancy behaves as a dominant trait (4,55). Similar conclusions were reached by others using polyoma virus-transformed mouse cells as the malignant parent (16); however, Harris et al. (28), Klein et al. (32), and Wiener et al. (75), based on an extensive study of a large number of mouse somatic cell hybrids, came to the opposite conclusion. In these studies, they showed that when highly malignant mouse cells were fused with normal mouse embryo cells, or mouse cells of low malignant potential, the resulting hybrids were transiently suppressed in their ability to form tumors (28,32,75). Tumorigenic segregants appeared with variable frequency (many of them very rapidly) in these nontumorigenic hybrid populations. Detailed analyses of the chromosome complements of the parental and hybrid cell populations indicated that the tumorigenic segregants had lost substantial numbers of chromosomes, including many of those originating from the normal parent. The interpretation of Harris and colleagues, that malignancy appears to behave as a recessive trait in somatic cell hybrids, has been supported by the studies of many other investigators using mouse, rat, and hamster intraspecies somatic cell hybrids (31,53) as well as interspecies rodent × human cell hybrids (12). However, there were notable exceptions to this generalization [reviewed in Croce (13)], particularly in the case where malignant cells that had been transformed by oncogenic viruses were used (14,15). The major drawback in virtually all of the studies described has been the chromosomal instability of the hybrid cells. Where a significant proportion of the total chromosome complement is rapidly lost, the chromosome loss may be random, as in the case of intraspecies rodent cell hybrids (42), or nonrandom, as in the case of human × rodent cell hybrids, where there is unidirectional segregation of human chromosomes (13). This rapid chromosome loss, in addition to making the initial premise of suppression of malignancy hard to evaluate, renders the identification of specific chromosomes that possibly control the expression of the tumorigenic phenotype an extremely arduous task. Approximately 10 years ago, Stanbridge (60) reexamined the question of the genetic control of malignancy by using intraspecies human cell hybrids. In this case (examined in more detail in the following sections), hybrid cells derived from the fusion of malignant HeLa cells with normal human diploid fibroblasts showed complete suppression of the tumorigenic phenotype (60). The suppression of malignancy was extremely stable, and tumorigenic segregants arose only rarely (63). Thus, this approach, using intraspecies human cell hybrids, generated a stable genetic model whereby one could look for the genetic factors that modulated malignant expression. The key to the stability of expression of the relevant phenotypic traits of these human somatic cell hybrids was their extreme chromosome stability.

TRANSFORMED AND TUMORIGENIC PHENOTYPES ARE UNDER SEPARATE GENETIC CONTROL

The early studies by Harris and colleagues clearly demonstrated that the mouse cell hybrids that were suppressed with respect to their tumorigenic potential still behaved as transformed cells in culture (27,69). This phenomenon of continued expresson of the transformed phenotype, concordant with the loss of the tumor-forming ability of hybrid cells, has been confirmed in virtually all somatic cell hybrid systems examined. In certain instances, however, somatic cell hybrids have been formed from the fusion of malignant × normal cells, or even malignant × malignant cells, which exhibit a limited proliferative lifespan (5,10,48).

The availability of paired combinations of hybrid cells (one transformed but nontumorigenic; the other transformed and tumorigenic) prompted the comparative analysis of their phenotypic characteristics. If we accept the position that the nontumorigenic hybrid cells are analogous to an intermediate step in the progression of a normal cell to a neoplastic cell (that is, a transformed nontumorigenic intermediate), then the comparative analysis of nontumorigenic hybrids and their tumorigenic segregants may allow us to determine which phenotypic traits are specifically correlated with tumorigenic expression. In many studies where markers of malignancy have been sought, they have been tentatively identified on the basis of comparisons between the neoplastic cells and their normal progenitor cells. The fact that the somatic cell hybrid system gives us an opportunity to compare a transformed but nontumorigenic cell with its closely related tumorigenic segregant would seem a more feasible approach toward identifying those phenotypic traits critical for the expression of tumorigenicity. Comparative studies of such hybrid cells quickly identified many so-called markers of malignancy as phenotypes expressed in both nontumorigenic and tumorigenic cell hybrids. Of the many phenotypic markers that would now seem to be associated with the transformed phenotype rather than the tumorigenic phenotype, perhaps the most surprising is that of anchorage independence. It has been repeatedly documented that the ability of cells to grow in suspension is correlated very strongly with tumorigenic expression (22,57). Although most of the studies have involved rodent cells, the dogma that anchorage-independent growth is synonymous with tumorigenicity has been extrapolated to other species, including human (26). Studies with both intraspecies rodent cell hybrids and intraspecies human cell hybrids indicate that this phenotype does not necessarily correlate specifically with tumorigenicity (although it may be a necessary alteration in the progression to malignancy, since many malignant cells express this trait), since many of the transformed nontumorigenic hybrid cells examined grow perfectly well in suspension in agarose or methyl cellulose (40,67).

Although nontumorigenic hybrid cells express many of the phenotypic traits of transformed cells in culture, some differences between nontumorigenic hybrid cells and their tumorigenic segregants have been documented. Documentation of such differences has been most extensive in intraspecies human cell hybrids, namely, HeLa × fibroblast hybrids. The first to be identified was an interesting integral membrane protein that is expressed by the parental HeLa population and tumorigenic segregant hybrids but not by fibroblasts or nontumorigenic hybrids. This marker is a 75-kilodalton (kD) glycophosphoprotein (Fig. 1), which migrates as a 150-kD dimer under nonreducing conditions (17). Further characterization of the purified material has revealed an associated protein kinase activity (70). This is a relatively unique tumor-associated marker, whose presence has been noted in only a few cancer cell lines of a large number tested (M. Greaves and E.J. Stanbridge, *unpublished observations*).

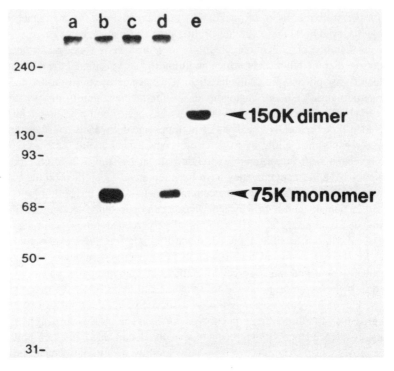

FIG. 1. Identification of a 75-kD tumor-associated antigen. Metabolically labeled cells were RIPA extracted and immunoprecipitated with anti-75-kD antibody: *(lane a)*, normal human fibroblasts; *(lane b)*, parental HeLa cells; *(lane c)*, nontumorigenic HeLa × fibroblast hybrid; *(lane d)*, tumorigenic segregant HeLa × fibroblast hybrid; *(lane e)*, nonreduced immunoprecipitate of lane d. (From ref. 17.)

A comparison of the properties of the 75-kD tumor-associated antigen and the human nerve growth factor (NGF) receptor (24) reveals very striking similarities (Table 1). Monoclonal antibodies against the 75-kD protein (6) immunoprecipitate a 75-kD protein from surface-labeled extracts of human melanoma cells expressing high levels of NGF receptor (E.J. Stanbridge, *unpublished observations*). Whether the two antigens recognized by this monoclonal antibody are the same protein or not must await further characterization.

Another tumor-associated antigen has been identified in HeLa × fibroblast hybrids and has been shown to have considerable promise for the clinical detection of malignancy within humans. This is the Ca antigen, described by Ashall and colleagues (1,9). A monoclonal antibody directed against Hep II cells—a possible HeLa contaminant—was found to react against HeLa and tumorigenic segregant hybrid cells, but not against fibroblasts or nontumorigenic hybrid cells. The antibody recognizes two components that separate in electrophoresis with apparent molecular weights of 390 and 350 kD. Subsequently, it was found that the antigen

TABLE 1. *Comparative properties of the 75-kD tumor-associated antigen and human nerve growth factor receptor*

Property	75-kD Tumor-associated protein[a]	Nerve growth factor receptor[b]
Apparent MW	70,000–75,000	70,000–75,000
Core protein MW	~60,000	59,000
Isoelectric point	Not determined	4.9–5.2
Glycosylation	N-linked	N-linked, possible O-linked
Phosphorylation	Serine-linked	Serine-linked
Kinase activity	Serine residues	Not determined

[a]Data from ref. 70.
[b]Data from ref. 24.

is present in a variety of cell lines derived from human cancers. More interesting, it was also found that the antibody reacted in immunohistochemical tests with a wide range of malignant human tumor cells in serous fluids (76). Further characterization of the antigen has shown it to be a highly glycosylated polypeptide with features of a mucin-like protein (9).

The final tumor-associated marker to be identified in HeLa × fibroblast hybrids was the ectopic expression of the α subunit of human chorionic gonadotrophin (HCG-α). Synthesis of HCG-α is absent or is at low basal levels in nontumorigenic hybrids, whereas it is expressed in moderate to high levels in all tumorigenic hybrids examined (66).

The functional significance of these tumor-associated markers in the expression of tumorigenicity in HeLa × fibroblast hybrids is at present unknown.

ASSOCIATION OF SPECIFIC CHROMOSOMES WITH SUPPRESSION OF MALIGNANCY

Great difficulties have been encountered in identifying specific chromosomes from the normal parent that may be involved in the suppression of tumorigenic phenotype in somatic cell hybrids. This is particularly true of intraspecies cell hybrids, where discrimination between chromosomes from normal versus malignant parental cells is extremely difficult. Several investigators have taken advantage of interspecies cell hybrids, particularly those of rodent × human hybrid cells, where there is unidirectional segregation of the human chromosomes. Also, the human chromosomes can be rather readily distinguished from the rodent complement. However, the problem with most of these studies is the rapidity of the loss of the human chromosomes. This loss can sometimes be so rapid that suppression of tumorigenicity is not seen. In other instances, the suppression may be only transient.

Very few of these studies have revealed the association of specific normal chromosomes with suppression of tumorigenicity; however, extensive studies by Klinger and collaborators (33,34), especially with hybrids between Chinese hamster tumorigenic cells and normal human fibroblasts, have provided evidence for the presence of tumor-suppressor genes on several human chromosomes. They found that the human chromosome 2 was not retained in any of the tumorigenic segregant hybrid cells examined and that chromosomes 9, 10, 11, and 17 were rarely present. In their careful analyses, they particularly examined for human chromosomes preferentially lost in pairwise combination. In addition to those chromosomes listed above, chromosomes 4, 7, 8, and 13 were detected as likely candidates for containing cosuppressor genes.

More recently, Stoler and Bouck (68) fused normal human fibroblasts to carcinogen-transformed baby hamster kidney (BHK) cells. In the hybrid cells formed, it was found that the anchorage-independent transformed phenotype was suppressed. Karyotype analysis indicated that only human chromosome 1 was retained in all hybrids that were suppressed and was lost in all hybrids in which the anchorage-independent phenotype was reexpressed (68). Clones reexpressing the anchorage-independent phenotype were isolated from two suppressed hybrids, and in both cases loss of suppression was accompanied by the loss of human chromosome 1. Although tumorigenicity was not assayed in these experiments, it had been shown previously that anchorage independence is highly correlated with the malignant phenotype in these particular hybrid cells.

In the earlier extensive studies of Harris, Klein, and colleagues (28,29,32,75), they were unable to establish the association of any particular chromosome with suppression of the tumorigenic phenotype. Although a role for chromosome 4 was suggested in certain of their studies, the authors felt that their evidence was not adequate (30). Subsequently, Harris and colleagues (19) reexamined the role of the normal chromosome 4 in the suppression of malignancy using natural polymorphisms of the centromeric heterochromatin to identify the parental origin of the chromosomes 4 in the hybrid cells. They found that the normal chromosome 4 was involved in the suppression of malignancy in all of the tumors that were examined, including carcinoma, melanoma, sarcoma, and lymphoma. In all crosses between malignant and normal cells there was a selective pressure *in vivo* against chromosome 4 derived from the normal cell and in favor of the chromosome 4 derived from the malignant cell. Thus, it would appear that chromosomes 4 in all tumors isolated were in some way functionally different from the chromosomes 4 of the normal parent. It was suggested that reappearance of malignancy in hybrids that were initially suppressed may result from a reduction in the number of copies of normal chromosome 4 and increase in the number of copies of malignant chromosome 4 or both. Thus, the gene or genes on the normal chromosome 4 responsible for the suppression of malignancy may act in a dose-dependent manner.

Sager and colleagues have undertaken an extensive analysis of intraspecies Chinese hamster hybrid cells [reviewed in Sager (52)]. Once again, the same phenomenon of suppression and reappearance of tumorigenic segregant hybrid cells was noted. Although extensive chromosome analyses were performed, no chromosomes have been identified that specifically correlate with suppression of the tumorigenic phenotype. The presence of a normal hamster chromosome 1 was associated with suppression of the anchorage-independent phenotype by Marshall and colleagues (40); however, in this case, this phenotype does not correlate with tumorigenic expression, and a number of anchorage-independent nontumorigenic hybrid clones were isolated. These results are therefore evidence of poor correlation between the loss of chromosome 1 and tumorigenicity.

The results with human intraspecies cell hybrids have been extremely consistent in the demonstration of suppression of tumorigenicity (33,63). Much of this work has been done using HeLa cells as the malignant parent and normal human diploid fibroblasts as the normal parent. Stanbridge and colleagues (65) described the loss of one copy each of two human chromosomes 11 and 14 associated with the reexpression of tumor-forming ability in HeLa × fibroblast hybrids. Klinger and associates (33), in a similar and very extensive study, also provided evidence supporting a role for human chromosome 11 in suppression of the tumorigenic phenotype. In their case, however, they also indicated that other human chromosomes, namely, 2, 13, 17, and 20, act as suppressors.

Benedict and colleagues (5) have analyzed paired combinations of nontumorigenic and tumorigenic segregant hybrids derived from the fusion of HT1080 human fibrosarcoma cells with human diploid fibroblasts. In this case, the loss of chromosome 1, and possibly chromosome 4, was associated with the restoration of tumorigenic potential in these hybrids. This is a particularly interesting result, since the N-*ras* oncogene, which is activated in HT1080 and in transfection experiments has been shown to transform mouse NIH3T3 cells (39), has been mapped to chromosome 1 (25). The possibility exists therefore that the chromosome 1 from the normal fibroblast may contain a gene that could not only suppress tumorigenic expression in the HT1080 × fibroblast hybrid but also regulate the expression of the activated N-*ras* gene if that gene is involved intrinsically in neoplastic expression.

The data derived from the HeLa and HT1080 hybrid cells clearly indicate that genes involved in controlling neoplastic expression in these two cancer cells are located on different chromosomes. This is not a surprising result, since the genes responsible for neoplastic expression in these two malignant cell types are likely to be different and therefore regulated by different *trans*-acting tumor-suppressor gene loci. It is worth noting that Weissman and Stanbridge (73) found that HeLa × HT1080 hybrid cells were nontumorigenic, indicating complementation of the malignant phenotype.

It should be emphasized that the cytogenetic analyses performed on the intraspecies human hybrid cells that implicate specific chromosomes in the control of expression of tumorigenicity can only be described as tentative. Unfortunately, due to the lack of morphologic markers identified by chromosome-banding techniques, it is impossible to determine the parental origin of those specific chromosomes that are absent in the tumorigenic segregants. The availability of chromosome-specific restriction-fragment-length polymorphism (RFLP) probes has now made it possible to identify specific chromosomes from different individuals (8,74) and thereby to ascertain the presence or absence of such chromosomes in somatic cell hybrids. Srivatsan and colleagues (59) have used this approach to analyze a series of intraspecies HeLa × fibroblast human cell hybrids, using RFLP probes specific for chromosomes 11 and 14. Loss of a single copy of these two chromosomes previously had been correlated with reexpression of tumorigenicity in HeLa × fibroblast hybrids using conventional cytogenetic banding techniques (65). The loss of a single copy of normal chromosome 11 from the hybrids was confirmed by RFLP analysis (Fig. 2), but no such correlation with loss of normal chromosome 14 was found (59). Far more extensive RFLP analyses will be required in order to determine whether tumor-suppressor genes capable of suppressing the tumorigenic phenotype in the HeLa × fibroblast hybrids reside on chromosome 11 alone or whether other cooperating tumor-suppressing genes are present on chromosomes other than 11 or 14.

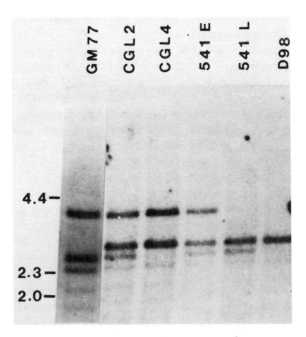

FIG. 2. RFLP analysis of parental and hybrid cells. Genomic DNAs of parental (GM77 and D98 are fibroblast and HeLa, respectively), nontumorigenic (CGL2 and 541E), and tumorigenic segregant (CGL4 and 541L) HeLa × fibroblast hybrids are digested with *TaqI* restriction endonuclease. DNA fragments were separated by electrophoresis on 0.8% agarose gels, transferred onto nitrocellulose filters and hybridized to a ^{32}P-labeled 6.6-kb c-Ha-*ras* probe. It is clearly seen that CGL 4 has lost the fibroblast 2.5-kb fragment and 541L has lost the fibroblast 4.0-kb fragment, thereby indicating in each case the loss of a fibroblast chromosome 11 in each of the tumorigenic hybrids. (From ref. 59.)

BIOLOGICAL NATURE OF SUPPRESSION OF TUMORIGENICITY

One of the general features of malignant × normal hybrid cell populations, whether interspecies human-rodent or intraspecies rodent or human hybrid populations, is that they behave as transformed cells in culture. An intriguing question therefore is why the nontumorigenic hybrids fail to form tumors in immunosuppressed mice when the growth behavior in culture is almost identical to that seen with the tumorigenic segregant hybrid populations. This question has really only been examined in detail with intraspecies human cell hybrids. Stanbridge and colleagues (62) noted that when nontumorigenic HeLa × fibroblast hybrid cells were inoculated subcutaneously into athymic mice, the cells initially proliferated, as if they would form tumors. However, approximately 4 days postinoculation, there was a dramatic decrease in mitotic activity. By day 7, virtually all mitotic activity had ceased, and the cells underwent a morphological alteration to a more fibroblastoid morphology (62). There was no evidence of lymphoid cell infiltration, and the tissue nodules remained well vascularized. The nature of the mitotic shutdown of the nontumorigenic hybrid cells in the mice remained enigmatic until a different set of hybrid cells were examined, namely, HeLa × keratinocyte hybrids. These hybrid cells have morphologic and growth properties similar to that of the HeLa parent (47). When the cells were inoculated subcutaneously into athymic mice, transient mitotic activity was seen for a number of days, and then gradual cessation of mitosis occurred. In the case of these hybrid cells, however, a very dramatic histological change is seen. The cells rather rapidly were induced to differentiate terminally. Most interesting, the nature of this terminal differentiation is that of keratinizing epithelium (47). Stanbridge and colleagues (64) have now accumulated considerable evidence to suggest that the nontumorigenic hybrid cells are induced to differentiate terminally in the athymic mouse and that the hybrid cell takes on the phenotypic signature of the normal parental cell, regardless of the origin of the malignant parental cell. For example, HeLa × keratinocyte hybrids differentiate into keratinocytes, and HeLa × fibroblast hybrids differentiate into fibroblasts in the intact animal. In all cases, the tumorigenic segregants of these hybrids form tumors that are undifferentiated anaplastic carcinomas, indistinguishable from those formed by the parental HeLa cells.

ONCOGENE EXPRESSION AND SUPPRESSION OF TUMORIGENICITY IN HYBRID CELLS

When the first oncogenes were discovered by DNA transfection studies in mouse NIH3T3 cells (37,49,56), there seemed to be a tacit assumption that a single, dominantly acting cellular gene was capable of transforming a cell into a cancerous state. This is a result that would be incompatible with both somatic cell hybridization data and epidemiological studies of human cancer. It was subsequently found that when primary or secondary cultures of rodent embryo cells were used in transfection assays, the cooperative action of two oncogenes was required to transform the cells (38,44). This multigenic interaction most closely approximates the conditions necessary for the multistage progression of cancer that has been evident from epidemiologic and experimental systems (3,20). Regardless of the number of oncogenes required, these and many other studies indicate that the cellular oncogenes are "dominantly acting." Equally clearly, most of the evidence from somatic cell hybrid experiments suggests that the tumorigenic phenotype can be suppressed by the introduction of normal genetic information. Thus, it is important to resolve the apparent paradox between "dominantly acting oncogenes" and "tumor-suppressor genes" capable of suppressing the tumorigenic phenotype. The extensive studies using HeLa as the malignant parental cell described above are uninformative in this regard, since no activated oncogene has been identified in this cell, and the DNA extracted from HeLa does not transform NIH3T3 cells in transfection assays. It should be noted, however, that O'Hara and colleagues (46) have reported that at least 11 proto-oncogenes are expressed in HeLa cells. The role of these expressed proto-oncogenes in contributing to the neoplastic phenotype of HeLa is unknown.

Two other hybrid cell combinations have been studied by Stanbridge and colleagues (5,23) that address this particular issue. The human fibrosarcoma cell line HT1080 contains an active N-*ras* gene capable of transforming mouse NIH3T3 cells (39). This cell line is also of interest because it is pseudodiploid but has a propensity to generate subtetraploid variants (5). It has been shown that the pseudodiploid HT1080 cell line is heterozygous at the N-*ras* locus, with the pseudodiploid cells containing one normal allele and one activated allele (7). Fusion of the pseudodiploid HT1080 cells with normal human diploid fibroblasts led to the isolation of hybrid cells that were tetraploid. These hybrid cells behaved as transformed cells in culture but failed to form tumors in nude athymic mice (5). Tumorigenic segregants, which were isolated at later times, had fully regained their tumorigenic potential. Thus, this hybrid cell system behaves in a fashion very similar to that seen with HeLa × fibroblast hybrids. When subtetraploid variants of HT1080 were fused with diploid fibroblasts, all of the near-hexaploid hybrid cell clones were as tumorigenic as the HT1080 parental cell. Thus, it would seem that tumorigenicity in this system appears to be chromosome-dose dependent. All hybrid cells that contained approximately twice the chromosome complement of the tumorigenic HT1080 parent were all highly tumorigenic, whereas the cell hybrids that contained approximately equal chromosomal representation from both HT1080 and normal human fibroblast cells were nontumorigenic. It is interesting that the tumorigenic segregants of these latter cells appeared to have lost at least one copy of chromosome 1. The fact that the loss of chromosome 1 was correlated with the expression of tumorigenicity in these near-tetraploid hybrids is of particular interest. The N-*ras* oncogene of HT1080 has been mapped to chromosome 1 (25). It has been suggested by several investigators (51) that tumorigenicity results from the balance of expressor versus suppressor chromosomes. The results with the HT1080 fibrosarcoma cell line suggest that there may be a balance between chromosomes containing information for the expression of tumorigenicity and chromosomes that can suppress tumorigenicity.

Data from Marshall and colleagues (C. Marshall, *personal communications*) would tend to support this notion. They have found that the tumorigenic pseudo-diploid HT1080 fibrosarcoma cell line contains one mutated (active) allele of N-*ras* and one normal allele (7). Marshall selected flat "revertants" of HT1080 by low serum selection and found that the revertants failed to form tumors when inoculated into nude athymic mice. These nontumorigenic revertants were found to be tetraploid [a common occurrence in this cell line (see Benedict et al. (5)] but most interesting, the ratio of mutated to normal alleles of N-*ras* was found to be 1:3. Repeated inoculation of these revertant cells into nude mice resulted in occasional tumor formation. The HT1080 cells established in culture from these tumors represented tumorigenic "rerevertants." These rerevertants remained tetraploid, but now the ratio of mutated to normal alleles of N-*ras* had shifted to 2:2 or 3:1. These results are somewhat analogous to the expressor:suppressor balance of chromosomes theory put forward by Sachs and colleagues (50,51) a number of years ago to explain a similar phenomenon in cultured hamster fibroblasts. In the case of HT1080, however, there is the intriguing possibility that varying amounts of normal versus mutated product of the N-*ras* gene may play a role in the neoplastic expression of these cells.

The important question in both the HT1080 revertant cells and the nontumorigenic HT1080 × fibroblast hybrid cells is whether the suppression of the tumorigenic phenotype is correlated with extinction of mutant N-*ras* gene expression. Weissman and colleagues (72) examined the possibility by immunoprecipitating the p21 protein product of the N-*ras* gene from nontumorigenic HT1080 × fibroblast hybrids with monoclonal antibodies. The striking and rather surprising result was that the level of expression of the p21 product was the same in both nontumorigenic and tumorigenic segregant hybrid cell populations (72). Thus, it would seem that suppression of the tumorigenic phenotype has occurred in the presence of continued expression of the N-*ras* oncogene. However, in these experiments, it was not possible to separate active from normal p21 product; therefore, it is possible that nontumorigenic and tumorigenic segregant HT1080 × fibroblast hybrid cells express high levels of normal versus active p21, respectively.

In a similar set of experiments, the human bladder carcinoma cell line EJ, which contains an activated c-Ha-*ras* gene was fused with normal human diploid fibroblasts. The DNA extracted from EJ cells is capable of transforming mouse NIH3T3 cells in a transfection assay. In these experiments, all of the EJ × fibroblast hybrid cells studied failed to form tumors in athymic mice, although the cells behaved like transformed cells in culture (23). Tumorigenic segregants were isolated from the suppressed hybrids that had regained full tumorigenic potential. These hybrid cells were examined for expression of the product of the c-Ha-*ras* gene (again, a p21 protein), both at the messenger RNA level via Northern blot analysis and by immunoprecipitation of the p21 protein. A similar result was found, namely, that the nontumorigenic and tumorigenic segregant hybrid cells express the same level of p21 protein (Figs. 3 and 4). In this case, because the p21 protein product of the activated allele of c-Ha-*ras* migrates more slowly than that of the normal p21 protein in polyacrylamide gels, it was possible to confirm that the high expression of p21 was that of the activated gene product. Further gene copies of the activated c-Ha-*ras* were transfected into the nontumorigenic EJ × fibroblast cells to see whether an enhanced expression of the activated p21 protein would lead to tumorigenic expression. Again, all the hybrids containing multiple copies of the activated c-Ha-*ras* gene remained nontumorigenic in spite of the elevated expression of p21. Thus, suppression of the tumorigenic phenotype was accomplished in the presence of continued expression of the activated c-Ha-*ras* oncogene.

There could obviously be a number of explanations for these results; however, a very likely explanation is that although the activated *ras* oncogenes seem to be late acting and their products crucial for neoplastic expression of transfected mouse cells, their expression in human somatic cell hybrids, although dominant, is insufficient to endow the cells with tumor-forming ability. This is not to suggest that the activated *ras* oncogenes play no role in the progression to tumorigenicity of the HT1080 fibrosarcoma and the EJ bladder carcinoma. It should be remembered that the nontumorigenic hybrid cells still behave like transformed cells in culture. Thus, in the cancer cells, where these activated oncogenes originate, they may play a role in some earlier stage of neoplastic progression.

The phenomenon of suppression of tumorigenicity with continued expression of an activated oncogene has also been documented in hamster cell hybrids, where the malignant parental cell was a Chinese hamster fibroblast transfected with the EJ c-Ha-*ras* oncogene (61). Also, nontumorigenic revertants of mouse fibroblasts transformed with Kirsten murine sarcoma virus continue to express the viral oncogene (45; see Bassin, *this volume*).

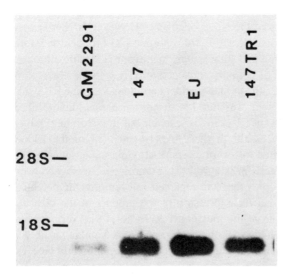

FIG. 3. Northern blot analysis of c-Ha-*ras* mRNA levels of fibroblast (GM2291 and EJ) bladder carcinoma parental cells and a representative nontumorigenic (147) and tumorigenic segregant EJ × fibroblast hybrid. The mRNA on the nitrocellulose filter was hybridized with a ³²P-labeled 2.2-kb fragment of c-Ha-*ras*. Shown are the 1.2-kb bands of c-Ha-*ras* messenger RNA. (From ref. 23.)

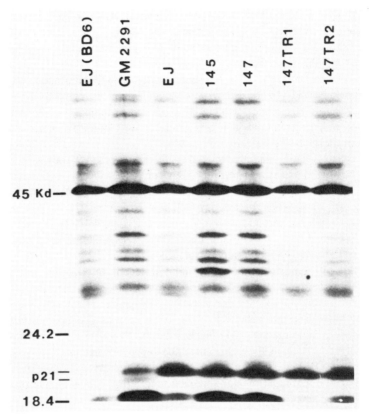

FIG. 4. SDS acrylamide gel analysis of c-Ha-*ras* p21 protein levels in parental and hybrid cells. The cells were metabolically labeled with [³⁵S]methionine, solubilized, and the extracts immunoprecipitated with an anti-p21 *ras* monoclonal antibody (YAC172). The immunoprecipitates were electrophoresed on a gradient SDS polyacrylamide gel. The gel was then dried and placed onto X-ray film. The locations of the immunoprecipitated p21 proteins are indicated on the *left*. The normal c-Ha-*ras* p21 protein seen in the fibroblast parent (GM2291) migrates more rapidly in the gel than the mutated EJ c-Ha-*ras*. The upper p21 band seen in GM2291 is the p21 product of c-Ki-*ras*, which is also recognized by the monoclonal antibody. The gel shows that approximately equal levels of activated p21 protein are expressed in the EJ parental cells, nontumorigenic (145,147), and tumorigenic segregant (147TR1, 147TR2) EJ × fibroblast hybrid cells. (From ref. 23.)

MOLECULAR APPROACHES TO IDENTIFYING TUMOR-SUPPRESSOR GENES

Studies involving intraspecies rodent, interspecies human-rodent, and intraspecies human somatic cell hybrids have shown in the majority of cases that tumorigenicity is suppressed when a cancer cell is fused with a normal cell. Some progress has been made in determining those chromosomes that may be involved in the control of tumorigenic expression and that therefore may contain tumor-suppressor gene loci (61). By its very nature, however, this approach to somatic cell hybridization, involving complete mammalian genomes, is a very crude genetic analysis, although it has proven to be useful in beginning to understand the genetic control of malignancy.

Dominantly acting oncogenes that score positively in transformation assays such as the mouse NIH3T3 system are readily recognized by searching for foci of multi-layered transformed cells on a monolayer of contact-inhibited cells. Appropriate molecular genetic techniques are then available for cloning the transfected onco-gene from the transformed cells (37,49,56).

The task of isolating and characterizing tumor-suppressor genes is by no means as straightforward as the transforming assay for oncogenes. By extrapolation from somatic cell hybridization studies, in the search for sequences that suppress tumor-igenicity we are looking for the rare cell that is nontumorigenic but *still trans-formed* against a background of transformed, tumorigenic cells. To achieve this, we will presumably require an indirect dominant selectable marker linked in some fashion to the putative tumor-suppressor gene.

One way to diminish the amount of normal genetic information transferred via cell fusion is to transfer single, specific normal chromosomes to the cancer cell. Two experimental approaches are possible. Metaphase chromosomes can be iso-lated and introduced into cells. This method has been used to successfully transfer dominant selectable markers (41) but has the disadvantage that the chromosomes are rapidly degraded in the cell. Thus, the procedure becomes, in a sense, the equivalent of DNA transfection, except that larger subchromosomal fragments are retained. The other experimental approach is to utilize the technique of microcell transfer where single chromosomes are transferred from donor to recipient cell in interphase micronuclei via cell fusion (18,21). This method has the advantage that the transferred chromosome is retained in the recipient cell in a heritable fashion and maintains its chromosome structural integrity. However, the problems of se-lection of the microcell hybrid and retention of the single human chromosome are in principle the same as those facing investigators who generate whole-cell hy-brids; that is, only a few chromosomes (e.g., the X chromosome) can be readily selected for and retained by use of selective media. This problem has now been circumvented by inserting dominant selectable markers into individual chromo-somes via DNA transfection (54,71). This approach has initially been used in pre-paring panels of microcell hybrids consisting of rodent cells containing single se-lectable human chromosomes that represent the entire human karyotype (P.J. Saxon and E.J. Stanbridge, *unpublished data*). Thus, any single human chromo-some may be transferred from donor microcell hybrid to recipient cancer or normal cell and its effect on the expression of the transformed or tumorigenic phenotype measured. Further refinements will include transfer of subchromosomal fragments of specific chromosomes, containing the selectable marker, that have been gener-ated by treating the microcell hybrid with chromosome-fragmenting chemicals or radiation. This methodology should allow us to localize more precisely genetic loci responsible for tumor suppression on chromosomes and eventually lead to successful cloning of these genes.

In studies reported in detail elsewhere in this volume (R.H. Bassin and M. Noda, *this volume*), other investigators have apparently suppressed the tumorigenic phenotype of Kirsten murine sarcoma-transformed mouse cells by DNA transfection by using DNA extracted from nontumorigenic flat revertants of the same cells. The revertant phenotype is associated with ouabain resistance (45) and is linked to altered expression of tropomyosin (11). The relationship of this effect to the tumor-suppressing effect seen in somatic cell hybrids remains to be determined.

ONCOGENES AND TUMOR-SUPPRESSOR GENES IN NATURALLY OCCURRING CANCERS

Both DNA transfection of human oncogenes into rodent cells and somatic cell hybridization experiments are artifactual in nature. It is therefore pertinent to ask if there is evidence for a direct role of activated oncogenes or tumor-suppressor genes in human cancer. The answer is yes in both cases. Many investigators have now examined a large number of human tumors for evidence of oncogene activation. In approximately 10% to 20% of tumors examined, mutated oncogenes, overexpressed oncogene products, or translocated oncogenes have been noted. Oncogene expression has been seen to occur in both early and late stages of malignancy (2).

There is evidence that a second group of genes, the "tumor-suppressor" genes (61) or "antioncogenes" of Knudson (35), are implicated in the genesis of human tumors. The most extensively studied examples are retinoblastoma and Wilm's tumor, respectively (36,43). Their detection was made possible by a combination of familial studies, cytogenetics, and molecular genetics involving particularly RFLP analyses. These tumor-suppressor genes may represent a class different from those identified in somatic cell hybrids, since they presumably represent genes that have an influence on the earliest events leading to malignant expression, whereas those suppressor elements identified in somatic cell hybrids represent control of expression of a late event (i.e., post-transformation) and possibly act on the ultimate event necessary for tumorigenic expression.

CONCLUSION

The phenomenon of tumor suppression measured in somatic cell hybrids has moved from a highly controversial area to a generally accepted fact. It would be naive to expect that the tumorigenic phenotype of all cancer cells will behave in a recessive manner and be suppressed by the introduction of genetic information from normal cells. However, this can occur with many cancer cells, including those that express apparently dominantly acting oncogenes. Methods are now available to proceed with the molecular characterization of tumor-suppressor genes. When this is accomplished, it should lead to a better understanding of the molecular basis of cancer and possibly lead to the identification of recessive onco-genes that may play an important role in the neoplastic process.

ACKNOWLEDGMENTS

The author's studies reported here were supported by grants from the National Cancer Institute (CA19401 and CA34114) and the Council for Tobacco Research-U.S.A. (No. 1475) and gifts from the Philip and Clarisse Fay Fund.

REFERENCES

1. Ashall, F., Bramwell, M.E., and Harris, H. (1982). A new marker for human cancer cells. 1. The Ca antigen and the Ca 1 antibody. *Lancet,* 2:1–6.
2. Balmain, A. (1985): Transforming *ras* oncogenes and multistage carcinogenesis. *Br. J. Cancer,* 51:1–8.
3. Barrett, J.C., and Ts'o, P.O.P. (1978): Evidence for the progressive nature of neoplastic transformation in vitro. *Proc. Natl. Acad. Sci. U.S.A.,* 75:3761–3765.
4. Barski, G., and Cornefert, F. (1962): Characteristics of "hybrid"-type clonal cell lines obtained from mixed cultures *in vitro. J. Natl. Cancer Inst.,* 28:801–821.
5. Benedict, W.F., Weissman, B.E., Mark, C., and Stanbridge, E.J. (1984): Tumorigenicity of human HT1080 fibrosarcoma × normal fibroblast hybrids is chromosome dosage dependent. *Cancer Res.,* 44:3471–3479.
6. Bicknell, D.C., Sutherland, D.R., Stanbridge, E.J., and Greaves, M.F. (1985): Monoclonal antibodies specific for a tumor-associated membrane phosphoprotein in human cell hybrids. *Hybridoma,* 4:143–152.
7. Bos, J.L., Verlaan de Vries, M., Veenemen, G.H., van Boom, A.J., and van der Eb. (1984): Three different mutations in codon 61 of the human N-*ras* gene detected by synthetic oligonucleotide hybridization. *Nucleic Acids Res.* 12:9155–9163.
8. Botstein, D., White, R., Skolnick, M., and Davis, R.W. (1980): Construction of a genetic linkage map in man using restriction-fragment-length polymorphisms. *Am. J. Hum. Genet.,* 32:314–331.
9. Bramwell, M.E., Bhavanandan, V.P., Wiseman, G., and Harris, H. (1983): Structure and function of the Ca antigen. *Br. J. Cancer,* 48:177–183.
10. Bunn, C.L., and Tarrant, G.M. (1980): Limited lifespan in somatic cell hybrids and cybrids. *Exp. Cell Res.,* 127:385–396.
11. Cooper, H.L., Feurstein, N., Noda, H., and Bassin, R.H. (1985): Suppression of tropomyosin synthesis—A common biochemical feature of oncogenesis by structurally diverse retroviral oncogenes. *Mol. Cell. Biol.,* 5:972–983.
12. Craig, R.W., and Sager, R. (1985): Suppression of tumorigenicity in hybrids of normal and oncogene-transformed CHEF cells. *Proc. Natl. Acad. Sci. U.S.A.,* 82:2062–2066.
13. Croce, C.M., (1984): Gene regulation in the expression of malignancy. *Cancer Surveys,* 3:287–298.
14. Croce, C.M., Aden, D., and Koprowski, H. (1975): Tumorigenicity of mouse-human diploid hybrids in nude mice. *Science,* 190:1200–1202.
15. Croce, C.M., and Koprowski, H. (1974): Somatic cell hybrids between peritoneal mouse macrophages and SV40-transformed human cells. I. Positive control of the transformed phenotype by the human chromosome 7 carrying the SV 40 genome. *J. Exp. Med.,* 140:1221–1229.
16. Defendi, V., Ephrussi, B., Koprowski, H., and Yoshida, M.C. (1967): Properties of hybrids between polyoma-transformed and normal mouse cells. *Proc. Natl. Acad. Sci. U.S.A.,* 57:299–305.

17. Der, C.J., and Stanbridge, E.J. (1981): A tumour-specific membrane phosphoprotein marker in human cell hybrids. *Cell,* 26:429–438.
18. Ege, T., Ringertz, N.R., Hamberg, H., and Sidebottom, E. (1977): Preparation of microcells. *Methods Cell Biol.,* 15:339–357.
19. Evans, E.P., Burtenshaw, M.D., Brown, B.B., Hennion, R., and Harris, H. (1982): The analysis of malignancy by cell fusion. IX. Reexamination and clarification of the cytogenetic problem. *J. Cell Sci.,* 56:113–130.
20. Foulds, L. (1975): *Neoplastic Development.* Academic Press, New York.
21. Fournier, R.E.K., and Ruddle, F.H. (1977): Microcell-mediated transfer of murine chromosomes into mouse, Chinese hamster, and human somatic cells. *Proc. Natl. Acad. Sci. U.S.A.,* 74:319–323.
22. Freedman, V.H., and Shin, S. (1974): Cellular tumorigenicity in nude mice: Correlation with cell growth in semisolid medium. *Cell,* 3:355–359.
23. Geiser, A., Der, C.J., Marshall, C.J., and Stanbridge, E.J. (1986): Suppression of tumorigenicity with continued expression of the c-Ha-*ras* oncogene in EJ bladder carcinoma × human fibroblast hybrid cells. *Proc. Natl. Acad. Sci. U.S.A.,* 83:5209–5213.
24. Grob, P.M., Ross, A.H., Koprowski, H., and Bothwell, M. (1985): Characterization of the human melanoma nerve growth factor receptor. *J. Biol. Chem.,* 260:8044–8049.
25. Hall, A., Marshall, C.J., Spurr, N.K., and Weiss, R.A. (1983): Identification of the transforming gene in two human sarcoma cell lines as a new member of the *ras* gene family located on chromosome 1. *Nature,* 303:316–400.
26. Hamburger, A.W., and Salmon, S.E. (1977): Primary bioessay of human tumor stem cells. *Science,* 197:461–463.
27. Harris, H. (1971): Cell fusion and the analysis of malignancy: The Croonian lecture. *Proc. Soc. Lond. [Biol.],* 179:1–20.
28. Harris, H., Miller, O.J., Klein, G., Worst, P., and Tachibana, T. (1969): *Nature,* 223:363–368.
29. Jonasson, J., and Harris, H. (1977): The analysis of malignancy by cell fusion. VIII. Evidence for the intervention of an extrachromosomal element. *J. Cell Sci.,* 24:255–263.
30. Jonasson, J., Povey, S., and Harris, H. (1977): The analysis of malignancy by cell fusion VII. Cytogenetic analysis of hybrids between malignant and diploid cells and of tumours derived from them. *J. Cell Sci.,* 24:217–254.
31. Kao, F., and Hartz, J.A. (1977): Genetic and tumorigenic characteristics of cell hybrids formed *in vivo* between injected tumor cells and host cells. *J. Natl. Cancer Inst.,* 59:409–413.
32. Klein, G., Bregula, U., Wiener, F., et al. (1971): The analysis of malignancy by cell fusion. I. Hybrids between tumour cells and L cell derivatives. *J. Cell Sci.,* 8:659–672.
33. Klinger, H.P. (1982): Suppression of tumorigenicity. *Cytogenet. Cell Genet.,* 32:68–84.
34. Klinger, H.P., and Shows, T.B. (1983): Suppression of tumorigenicity in somatic cell hybrids. II. Human chromosomes implicated as suppressors of tumorigenicity in hybrids with Chinese hamster ovary cells. *J. Natl. Cancer Inst.,* 79:559–569.
35. Knudson, A.G., Jr. (1985): Hereditary cancer, oncogenes, and antioncogenes. *Cancer Res.,* 45:1437–1443.
36. Koufos, A., Hansen, M.F., Lampkin, B.C., Workman, M.L., Copeland, N.G., Jenkins, N.A., and Cavenee, W.K. (1984): Loss of alleles at loci on human chromosome 11 during genesis of Wilm's tumour. *Nature,* 309:170–172.
37. Krontiris, T.G., and Cooper, G.M. (1981): Transforming activity of human tumour DNAs. *Proc. Natl. Acad. Sci. U.S.A.,* 78:1181–1184.
38. Land, H., Parada, L.F., and Weinberg, R.A. (1983): Tumorigenic conversion of primary embryo fibroblasts requires at least two cooperating oncogenes. *Nature,* 304:596–602.
39. Marshall, C.J., Hall, A., and Weiss, R.A. (1982): A transforming gene present in human sarcoma cell lines. *Nature,* 299:171–173.
40. Marshall, C.J., Kitchin, R.M., and Sager, R. (1982): Genetic analysis of tumorigenesis: XII. Genetic control of the anchorage requirement in CHEF cells. *Somatic Cell Mol. Genet.,* 8:709–721.
41. McBride, O.W., and H.L. Ozer. (1973): Transfer of genetic information by purified metaphase chromosomes. *Proc. Natl. Acad. Sci. U.S.A.,* 70:1258–1262.
42. Miller, D.A., and Miller, O.J. (1983): Chromosomes and cancer in the mouse: Studies in tumours, established cell lines, and cell hybrids. *Adv. Cancer Res.,* 39:153–182.
43. Murphree, A.L., and Benedict, W.F. (1984): Retinoblastoma: Clues to human oncogenesis. *Science,* 223:1028–1033.

44. Newbold, R.F., and Overell, R.W. (1983): Fibroblast immortality is a prerequisite for transformation by EJ c-Ha-*ras* oncogene. *Nature,* 304:648–651.
45. Noda, M., Selinger, Z., Scolnick, E.M., and Bassin, R.H. (1983): Flat revertants isolated from Kirsten sarcoma virus-transformed cells are resistant to the action of specific oncogenes. *Proc. Natl. Acad. Sci. U.S.A.,* 80:5602–5605.
46. O'Hara, B.M., Klinger, H.P., and Blair, D.G. (1985): *Fos* expression correlates with tumorigenicity in hybrids of HeLa and normal human fibroblasts. *First Ann. Meet. Oncogenes,* p. 67.
47. Peehl, D.M., and Stanbridge, E.J. (1982): The role of differentiation in the control of tumorigenic expression in human cell hybrids. *Intl. J. Cancer,* 30:113–120.
48. Pereira-Smith, O.M., and Smith, J.R. (1981): Expression of SV40T antigen in finite life span hybrids of normal and SV40-transformed fibroblasts. *Somatic Cell Mol. Genet.,* 7:411–421.
49. Perucho, M., Goldfarb, M., Shimizu, K., Lama, C., Fogh, J., and Wigler, M. (1981): Human tumour-derived cell lines contain common and different transforming genes. *Cell,* 27:467–476.
50. Rabinowitz, Z., and Sachs, L. (1968): Reversion of properties in cells transformed by polyoma virus. *Nature,* 220:1203–1206.
51. Sachs, L. (1984): Normal regulators, oncogenes, and the reversibility of malignancy. *Cancer Surveys,* 3:219–228.
52. Sager, R. (1985): Genetic suppression of tumor formation. *Adv. Cancer Res.,* 44:43–68.
53. Sager, R., and Kovac, P.E. (1978): Genetic analysis of tumorigenesis. I. Expression of tumor-forming ability in hamster hybrid cell lines. *Somatic Cell Mol. Genet.,* 4:375–392.
54. Saxon, P.J., Srivatsan, E.S., Leipzig, G.V., Sameshima, J.H., and Stanbridge, E.J. (1985): Selective tranfer of individual human chromosomes to recipient cells. *Mol. Cell. Biol.,* 5:140–146.
55. Scaletta, L.J., and Ephrussi, B. (1965): Hybridization of normal and neoplastic cells in vitro. *Nature,* 205:1169–1171.
56. Shih, C., Padhy, L.C., Murray, M., and Weinberg, R.A. (1981): Transforming genes of carcinomas and neuroblastomas introduced into mouse fibroblasts. *Nature,* 290:261–264.
57. Shin, S., Freedman, V.H., Risser, R., and Pollock, R. (1975): Tumorigenicity of virus-transformed cells in nude mice is correlated specifically with anchorage-independent growth *in vitro. Proc. Natl. Acad. Sci. U.S.A.,* 72:4435–4439.
58. Smith, B.L., and Sager, R. (1982): Multistep origin of tumor-forming ability in CHEF cells. *Cancer Res.,* 42:389–396.
59. Srivatsan, E.S., Benedict, W.F., and Stanbridge, E.J. (1986): Molecular analysis of the chromosomal control of neoplastic expression in human cell hybrids: Chromosome 11 is implicated in the suppression of tumorigenicity. *(Submitted.)*
60. Stanbridge, E.J. (1976): Suppression of malignancy in human cells. *Nature,* 260:17–20.
61. Stanbridge, E.J. (1985): A case for human tumor-suppressor genes. *Bioessays,* 3:252–255.
62. Stanbridge, E.J., and Ceredig, R. (1981): Growth regulatory control of human cell hybrids in nude mice. *Cancer Res.,* 41:573–580.
63. Stanbridge, E.J., Der, C.J., Doersen, C.J., Nishimi, R.Y., Peehl, D.M., Weissman, B.E., and Wilkinson, J. (1982): Human cell hybrids: Analysis of transformation and tumorigenicity. *Science,* 215:252–259.
64. Stanbridge, E.J., Fagg, B.A., and Der, C.J. (1983): Differentiation and the control of tumorigenicity in human cell hybrids. In: *Human Carcinogenesis,* edited by C. Harris and H. Autrup, pp. 97–122. Academic Press, New York.
65. Stanbridge, E.J., Flandermeyer, R.R., Daniels, D.W., and Nelson-Rees, W.A. (1981): Specific chromosome loss associated with the expression of tumorigenicity in human cell hybrids. *Somatic Cell Mol. Genet.,* 7:699–712.
66. Stanbridge, E.J., Rosen, S.W., and Sussman, H.H. (1982): Expression of the alpha subunit of human chorionic gonadotropin is specifically correlated with tumorigenic expression in human cell hybrids. *Proc. Natl. Acad. Sci. U.S.A.,* 79:6242–6245.
67. Stanbridge, E.J., and Wilkinson, J. (1980): Dissociation of anchorage independence from tumorigenicity in human cell hybrids. *Intl. J. Cancer,* 26:1–8.
68. Stoler, A., and Bouck, N. (1985): Identification of a single chromosome in the normal human genome essential for suppression of hamster cell transformation. *Proc. Natl. Acad. Sci. U.S.A.,* 80:570–574.
69. Straus, D.S., Jonasson, J., and Harris, H. (1976): Growth *in vitro* of tumour cell × fibroblast hybrids in which malignancy is suppressed. *J. Cell Sci.,* 25:73–86.
70. Sutherland, D.R., Bicknell, D.C. Downward, J., Parker, P., Baker, M.A., Greaves, M.F., and Stanbridge, E.J. (1986): Structural and functional features of a cell-surface phosphoglycoprotein

associated with tumorigenic phenotype in human fibroblast × HeLa cell hybrids. *J. Biol. Chem.,* 261:2418–2424.

71. Tunnacliffe, A., Parkar, M., Povey, S., Bengtsson, B.O., Stanley, K., Solomon, E., and Good-fellow, P. (1983): Integration of *Eco-gpt* and SV40 early-region sequences into human chromosome 17: A dominant selection system in whole-cell and microcell human-mouse hybrids. *EMBO J.,* 2:1577–1584.

72. Weissman, B.E., Mark, C.S., Benedict, W.F., and Stanbridge, E.J. (1985): Expression of the N-*ras* oncogene in tumorigenic and nontumorigenic HT1080 fibrosarcoma × normal human fibroblast hybrid cells. In: *Advances in Neuroblastoma Research,* edited by A.E. Evan, G.J. D'Angio, and R.C. Seeger, 175:141–149. Alan R. Liss, New York.

73. Weissman, B.E., and Stanbridge, E.J. (1983): Complementation of the tumorigenic phenotype in human cell hybrids. *J. Natl. Cancer Inst.,* 70:667–672.

74. White, R., Leppert, M., Bishop, D.T., Barker, D., Berkowitz, J., Brown, C., Callahan, P., Holm, T., and Jerominski, L. (1985): Construction of linkage maps with DNA markers for human chromosomes. *Nature,* 313:101–105.

75. Wiener, F., Klein, G., and Harris, H. (1974): The analysis of malignancy by cell fusion. V. Further evidence of the ability of normal diploid cells to suppress malignancy. *J. Cell Sci.,* 15:177–183.

76. Woods, J.C., Spriggs, A.I., Harris, H., and McGee, J.O'D. (1982): A new marker for human cancer cells. 3. Immunocytochemical detection of malignant cells in serous fluids with the Ca 1 antibody. *Lancet,* 2:512–515.

Advances in Viral Oncology, Volume 6, edited by
George Klein, Raven Press, New York © 1987.

Oncogene Inhibition by Cellular Genes

*Robert H. Bassin and **Makoto Noda

*Laboratory of Tumor Immunology and Biology, National Cancer Institute, Bethesda,
Maryland 20892; **The Institute of Physical and Chemical Research, Wako, Saitama,
351-01, Japan*

The rapid pace of current biological research, generated to a large degree by major technical and conceptual advances in molecular biology, is now resulting in significant progress toward an understanding of the fundamental biochemical mechanisms involved in tumor formation *in vivo* and in the related phenomenon of cell transformation *in vitro*. Nowhere has this progress been more evident than in the area of cell transformation by specific retroviral genes (oncogenes) and the significance of the normal cellular genes (proto-oncogenes) from which they derive (4–6). In many cases, individual oncogenes responsible for one or more of the phenomena associated with tumor formation and cell transformation have been identified and their molecular structures solved.

In contrast to advances in the identification and characterization of the structural relationships of oncogenes (and their products) to one another and to normal cellular components, the specific molecular mechanisms by which oncogenes transform cells have yet to be determined. Although it is known that transformed cells differ from their nontransformed progenitors in many biological and biochemical properties, those critical functions, without which transformation cannot occur, remain obscure. Moreover, tumor formation in the animal host seems to involve an even greater complexity of molecular changes than does cell transformation *in vitro* (44,48,52,97).

One approach to understanding the mechanisms of cell transformation involves the isolation and analysis of genotypically altered cells possessing changes in the critical biochemical pathways by which transformation is effected. Some of these cells may be altered in such a way as to render them resistant to transformation by one or more specific oncogenes. The analysis of such cells could result not only in the identification of molecular mechanisms essential for induction of the transformed phenotype but also in the characterization of cellular products or other agents capable of preventing or even reversing the transformation process (18,34,71–73).

This review discusses evidence for the existence and behavior of cells genetically resistant to transformation by specific oncogenes. The isolation and characterization of cells resistant to the action of retroviral oncogenes is emphasized. In the following discussion, we shall use the term "oncogene" to describe any DNA sequence that may be considered directly or indirectly responsible for the induction of one or more characteristics of cell transformation. For simplicity, we shall consider the terms "cell transformation" and "tumor formation" to be interchangeable, even though the latter is in all likelihood a far more complex process of which the changes corresponding to cell transformation *in vitro* may be only one component.

NATURALLY OCCURRING RESISTANCE TO THE TRANSFORMED PHENOTYPE

The existence of naturally occurring genes that confer resistance to oncogenic agents is suggested by two kinds of data: (a) the behavior of certain human tumors, including retinoblastoma, Wilm's Tumor, neuroblastoma, and others whose occurrence involves the *loss* of specific DNA sequences; and (b) the analysis of hybrids generated by fusion of nontransformed and transformed cells to one another.

Retinoblastoma, for example, is known to occur in either a hereditary form (characterized by multifocal tumors, occurrence in younger patients, and by an increased susceptibility of the patient to other kinds of primary malignancies) or a nonhereditary form (characterized by unifocal tumors, occurrence in older patients, and by the absence of increased susceptibility to other kinds of malignancies. As reviewed by Murphree and Benedict (57) and by Knudson (46), the occurrence of retinoblastoma is controlled by a diploid pair of inhibitor alleles at the "retinoblastoma locus," Rb-1, located at 13q14, whose product may be a naturally-occurring cellular inhibitor of this malignancy. Alterations at the Rb-1 locus are recessive, and loss or inactivation of both alleles is presumed to be required for the development of a tumor. Thus, in the hereditary form of the disease, one defective copy of the Rb-1 locus is inherited, and the second copy is inactivated by an unknown mechanism, apparently involving a loss or rearrangement at location 13q14 in some cases and point mutations in others. In the nonhereditary form of retinoblastoma, both copies of the Rb-1 locus in a single somatic cell are inactivated, a much rarer event. The increased incidence of other types of tumors observed in the hereditary forms of retinoblastoma may indicate that the Rb-1 locus can control other potentially oncogenic genes. A molecular study (12) using probes to the 13q14 region has confirmed that in at least two cases of the hereditary form of the disease, a variant Rb-1 allele is indeed inherited from one parent, and a wild-type Rb-1 allele from the other parent. In the retinoblastoma cells themselves, the wild-type allele is no longer detectable. Although the mechanism by which normal alleles are able to suppress the occurrence of retinoblastomas and other kinds of heritable tumors is not yet known, the fact that repression is a dominant characteristic indicates that there is an active inhibition of the oncogene(s) responsible for tumor formation in these cases, perhaps mediated by some product of the Rb-1 allele. Studies with dominant suppression of the transformed phenotype by putative resistance genes in several tumor systems have been reviewed by Murphree and Benedict (57) and Knudson (46) and appear elsewhere in this volume.

The occurrence of cellular genes that inhibit transformation is also indicated in somatic cell hybridization experiments, where in certain cases, the nontransformed phenotype is dominant in hybrids between a nontransformed parent and a transformed parent (3,37,45,64,71–73,77,78,84,85). These studies have also been reviewed by Sager (71–73) and in the chapter by Stanbridge *(this volume)*. Most of the somatic cell hybridization studies have involved cells transformed by one or more undefined oncogenes, and the nature of the suppression is usually unknown.

Stoler and Bouck (88) have studied suppression of transformation by diploid human fibroblasts. In their studies, suppression was indicated by the loss of anchorage-independent growth in hybrids between normal human cells and the chemically transformed DMN 4A derivative of BHK 21/13 hamster cells. It had been shown previously that acquisition of the ability to grow in agar by the DMN 4A line, a property that correlates well with tumorigenicity, involves only a single mutagenic step (7,8). Studies on the detection, isolation, and characterization of a possible ''suppressor gene'' would seem to be much less difficult to interpret in this type of defined model. In fact, fusion of human fibroblasts to transformed DMN 4A cells resulted in hybrids that were unable to grow in agar suspension cultures, whereas hybrids between the same fibroblasts and SV40-transformed BHK cells showed a high colony-forming activity (88). Moreover, chromosomal analysis of the hybrid clones suggested that only human chromosome 1 is necessary for suppression of colony-forming activity in DMN 4A cells. It will be interesting to see if the particular DNA sequence responsible for suppression can be identified, perhaps by using DNA-mediated transfection techniques. These experimental results indicate the advantages of using cells transformed by single, definable genetic changes to detect and to characterize potential inhibitors of transformation. Cells transformed by retroviral oncogenes also fulfill these requirements. In fact, Dyson *et al.* (15,25–27,62,101,102) were able to show quite early that avian Rous sarcoma virus was unable to initiate transformation in rat cells with high efficiency because of a *trans*-acting cellular activity in these cells that inhibits transcription of the Rous sarcoma provirus.

Many acutely transforming retroviruses contain specific transforming oncogenes that are relatively easy to analyze and are capable of rapidly transforming cells *in vitro* or of inducing specific kinds of tumors in animals. The application of molecular techniques to studies on the mechanisms of transformation by individual retroviral oncogenes, as summarized in the next section, has resulted in an explosion of information concerning the genetic and biochemical changes involved in cell transformation. As a result, cells transformed by retroviral oncogenes promise to be useful reagents with which to identify genes and their products that are capable of interfering with the transformation process.

MOLECULAR ANALYSIS OF RETROVIRAL ONCOGENES

Retroviruses have long been used as convenient tools with which to examine the mechanism of transformation both *in vitro* and *in vivo* [see Weiss et al. (98) for review]. In addition to the suitability of retroviral oncogenes for studies on the inhibition of cell transformation mentioned above, other well-known advantages of using retroviruses in studies on cell transformation include (a) the rapid, direct, and reproducible nature of the changes induced by retroviral oncogenes; (b) the relatively high efficiency with which these oncogenes can be introduced into host cells; (c) the wide variety of animal species and cell types that are susceptible to transformation by retroviruses; and (d) the relative stability of the transformed phenotype as a result of covalent integration of the retroviral provirus into the genome of the host cell.

Molecular studies with various isolates of retroviruses indicate general similarities in structure. Retrovirus replicative cycles always involve a DNA intermediate (the provirus), which is usually inserted randomly into the host cell genome. From one group of retroviruses whose characteristics include rapid tumor induction *in vivo* and rapid transformation of appropriate cells in culture, some 30 different oncogenes have been identified. The protein products of these retroviral oncogenes appear to be required for expression and maintenance of the transformed phenotype. Each of these retroviral oncogenes is related, but not identical, to an endogenous cellular proto-oncogene from which the transforming retrovirus was generated. General reviews of retroviral oncogenes and proto-oncogenes have been published (4,5,98).

Many primary tumors and tumor cell lines, including those from humans, also contain DNA sequences, which on extraction and transfection into susceptible cells induce transformed foci and/or permit the cells to grow either in soft agar or as tumors in nude mice (21,31,65,76). In some cases, these human transforming sequences are derived from the same cellular proto-oncogenes and have similar sequence alterations as do the corresponding retroviral oncogenes. An example of this relationship was the isolation by the above procedures of transforming sequences from human bladder carcinoma cells (31,65,76). In this case, the sequences responsible for transformation were shown to be homologous to the v-Ha-*ras* gene and differed by as little as a single base change from the related normal cellular proto-oncogene. Thus, cellular proto-oncogenes are a source not only of the transducible oncogenes associated with retroviruses but also of additional oncogenes in tumor cells that may not be associated with retroviruses. Other transforming sequences which do not appear to have retroviral counterparts have been isolated from human tumors, [see Marshall (53) for review].

Sukumar et al. (89) have used the experimental model of nitrosomethylurea-induced mammary carcinomas in rats to investigate the role of proto-oncogenes in the induction of tumors *in vivo*. In this controlled experimental system, chemically induced malignancy can be correlated with the presence in the tumor cells of a single specific base change in the proto-oncogene c-Ha-*ras*.

Retroviral oncogenes, then, seem to represent the ideal agents with which to analyze the molecular and biochemical mechanisms of the transformation process and its inhibition. They are not only relatively easy to study in the laboratory, but are involved in the process of tumor formation in animals and man.

FUNCTIONS OF RETROVIRAL ONCOGENES AND THEIR PRODUCTS

A primary objective of studies on the resistance of cells to transformation by retroviral oncogenes is the identification of the pathways by which oncogenes induce the transformed phenotype. It is therefore important first to consider results of other kinds of studies that may relate the functions of oncogenes and their products to the mechanisms of transformation. There are several approaches to this problem that are already being exploited or that may be expected to yield useful information in the near future. Some of these studies are briefly outlined below.

Analysis of Proto-Oncogenes

As mentioned above, retroviral oncogenes are probably derived from normal cellular proto-oncogenes, which they closely resemble structurally. Proto-oncogene sequences are highly conserved phylogenetically. They are expressed in certain kinds of normal cells both *in vitro* and *in vivo*, and it is reasonable to assume that the proteins they encode are involved in fundamental cell processes (43,47,56). Analysis of the expression of these proto-oncogenes in various normal tissues may give important clues to the function of related retroviral oncogenes. For example, the proto-oncogenes c-*myc* and c-*myb* are preferentially expressed in hematopoietic cells; c-*abl* and c-*mos* in testes; and c-*src* in neuronal cells (43,56). Some proto-oncogenes appear to be regulated during development and differentiation (82,83,99); others appear to respond to events in the cell cycle (11).

Studies on the expression and other properties of proto-oncogenes must be interpreted carefully, however. There are various kinds of structural differences between the products of transforming retroviral oncogenes and those of the proto-oncogenes to which they are related (24). In addition to these structural differences, the transforming oncogenes found in retroviruses are under the transcriptional control of retrovirus promotor and enhancer sequences (98), and their expression patterns may differ both quantitatively and qualitatively from that of the original proto-oncogene. Also, some retroviruses contain two proto-oncogenes apparently working cooperatively to transform cells (see the chapter by Jansen and Bister, *in this volume*). Despite these differences, however, the functions of some retroviral oncogene products might be more or less the same as those encoded by structurally related proto-oncogenes. Transformation could then result either from the inappropriate expression of a proto-oncogene sequence under retroviral control (13) or from the synthesis of an altered gene product, which may or may not exhibit the same function as its homologous proto-oncogene. The expression of individual proto-oncogenes in various tissues, at various stages of embryogenesis, at different stages of the cell cycle, and in regenerating tissues is currently under intensive study (11,32,33,82,99,103).

Studies of Proto-Oncogenes in Lower Organisms

Homologs to the c-Ha-*ras* proto-oncogene have been detected and studied in eukaryotic species ranging from yeast to man (14,19,68). In *Escherichia coli*, amino acid sequence homologies between the Tu elongation factor, a GDP binding protein, and p21 have been reported (40). The yeast species *Saccharomyces cerevesiae* contains two 2 genes, *RAS*1 and *RAS*2, which are structurally related to the human proto-oncogenes c-Ha-*ras*-1 and c-Ha-*ras*-2 (19,68). Experiments with yeast are in many ways easier to perform and to analyze than experiments with mammalian cells, and it has already been determined that the yeast cell requires the functioning of at least one of its *RAS* genes for sporulation (42). Reports (9,90) have indicated that the yeast *RAS* gene product is concerned with the regulation of adenylate cyclase activity, but it is not clear that the *ras* gene performs the same function in mammalian cells (2). It is of interest, however, that the mammalian gene v-Ha-*ras* isolated from human cells can replace the requirement for *RAS*1 and *RAS*2 when introduced into the yeast cell (20,41). Studies with the mammalian proto-oncogenes c-*src* and c-*abl*, homologs of which are identifiable in *Drosophila* DNA, are also in progress. These and other studies designed to determine the functions of proto-oncogenes in lower organisms should be critical to a basic understanding of the mechanism of transformation in mammalian cells by retroviral oncogenes.

Molecular Analysis of Oncogenes and Their Products

Evidence regarding the possible functions of retroviral oncogenes and their products can be gained by comparing nucleic acid and protein sequence data to those of other known genes. The first example of this approach was the analysis of the v-*sis* gene product, p28, which was shown to be closely homologous to platelet-derived growth factor (PDGF) (22,96). A close relationship between the retroviral oncogene v-*erb*-B and the receptor for epidermal growth factor has been demonstrated at both the nucleic acid and protein levels (23,94). The product of another retroviral oncogene, v-*src*, appears to be closely related to the receptor for insulin, and antibodies against the v-*src* protein, pp60[v-*src*], precipitate insulin receptor protein (67,93). Analyses of nucleic acid and amino acid sequences from retroviral oncogenes have also shown similarities between members of the *ras* gene family and the Gproteins of the adenylate cyclase system (2). The product of the v-*fms* oncogene is a protein kinase and is related to the receptor for the growth factor CSF-1 (79).

In many cases, then, oncogenes appear to be related to growth factors or to growth factor receptors. Unfortunately, the biochemical pathways by which growth factors act are not well-understood at this time, but advances in this area will also help in elucidating the mechanism of transformation by at least some of the retroviral oncogenes. It is already clear, however, that many of the growth factor receptors function as tyrosine kinases and that this property may be the key to their activity (16,39). Moreover, other oncogene products possess tyrosine kinase activity but have not been shown to be related to any normal cellular protein (5).

Possible functions of the proteins encoded by the *ras* family of oncogenes are of special interest to this review, not only because transforming sequences related to *ras* are frequently isolated from human tumors (53), but also because many of the attempts to isolate cells resistant to transformation by oncogenes, as discussed below, have involved the *ras* gene and the *ras*-encoded transforming protein, p21. The product of the *c-ras* proto-oncogene, has been isolated from nontransformed mammalian cells and p21$^{c\text{-}ras}$, is a membrane-associated (100), GTP binding protein (80) with GTPase activity. The product of the v-*ras* oncogene, p21$^{v\text{-}ras}$, in addition, catalyzes autophosphorylation, but exhibits a reduced GTPase activity. Properties of the *ras* gene and its protein product have been reviewed by Shih and Weeks (81).

Besides analyses on a molecular level, immunological studies with proteins encoded by viral oncogenes have been used extensively to indicate their subcellular distribution, to detect protein kinase activities, and to indicate cellular proteins that may be specifically associated with oncogene products in cells (100). Newer technologies that permit the production of antisera and monoclonal antibodies against synthetic peptides should enhance the value of these experiments.

Another potentially valuable approach to gaining information concerning the function of retroviral oncogenes and their products involves studies on cells that are resistant to transformation by specific oncogenes. A detailed discussion of this area of research is the major subject of the remainder of this review.

CELLS RESISTANT TO TRANSFORMATION BY RETROVIRAL ONCOGENES

Strategies for the Isolation of Resistant Cells

The isolation and characterization at the molecular level of genetically altered cells that are resistant to transformation by one or more oncogenes has almost unlimited potential as a method for understanding not only the function of oncogenes and the cellular pathways with which they interact but also for indicating procedures by which the transformation process can be reversed. The advent of recombinant DNA techniques, including site-specific mutagenesis, renders such a genetic approach even more practical. However, progress in this area has until recently been almost nonexistent, largely because of several technical problems encountered in the isolation of cells with the desired genotypes.

First, there has been no suitable selective system for identifying cells resistant to transformation in a parental population of *nontransformed* susceptible cells. Testing individual cells or clones of cells for resistance to transformation in the absence of some enrichment or selection procedure designed to increase the proportion of useful variants seems hopelessly difficult, and such a procedure has been eschewed by most investigators. (It should be noted, however, that with rapidly increasing knowledge of the nature and importance of growth factors in the transformation process, it should soon be possible to establish culture conditions whereby resistant cells that arise in populations of nontransformed cells may be recognized by their altered phenotypic responses to individual growth factors without direct challenge with transforming oncogenes).

An alternative strategy involves the isolation of transformation-resistant variants from parental populations of *transformed* cells. This strategy allows identification and selection of resistant cells simply by isolating clonal populations of morphologically nontransformed or "revertant" cells based on their appearance under the microscope. Although this type of procedure is not without its own problems (see below), it is the only strategy that has so far led to the isolation of cells resistant to specific oncogenes.

The frequency of occurrence of revertant cells resistant to transformation by specific oncogenes is unknown at this time. Moreover, since it is anticipated that changes in any one of several different cellular properties may be sufficient to render a cell resistant to one or more oncogenes, the frequency of each kind of revertant may be very low indeed. Selective procedures that may enrich the proportion of all nontransformed revertants or even of specific groups of revertants would be highly advantageous, and a second strategy to be employed in selecting cells resistant to transformation by oncogenes is the development and use of techniques that enrich the proportion of rare nontransformed cells in populations containing a vast excess of transformed cells. Our very rough estimates indicate that enrichments by factors of at least 10^3 to 10^4 are required. Selective inhibition of transformed cells in mixed populations containing nontransformed cells is difficult, since the transformed cell is endowed with additional growth potential under almost every known growth condition. Enrichment procedures used previously to select nontransformed cells in mixed populations usually have taken advantage of the ability of transformed cells to grow selectively in suspension cultures or in crowded monlayers. Such procedures, or "negative selection" techniques, require the addition of toxic agents such as BUdR or radioactively labeled thymidine under conditions that favor their incorporation by transformed cells (36). These techniques have been used successfully in at least two cases to isolate cells resistant to transformation (35,62), but the enrichment may not be sufficient to be used successfully on a routine basis.

New selective techniques may be required for the isolation of a comprehensive library of cells resistant to transformation. The use of ouabain as a selective inhibitor of *ras*-transformed revertant cells is described below. It is likely, however, that additional selective agents will be required in future. In fact, it may be possible to use different methods of selection to isolate different classes of resistant cells. Potential methods of selection include the use of the differential effect of methionine (38,69) and paraquat (28) on transformed versus control cells. The use of different substrates that selectively allow attachment of either transformed or nontransformed cells would seem to represent the ideal selective procedure, since it does not involve cell toxicity and could be used several times in succession to enrich populations and therefore has the potential of selecting cells that differ in attachment kinetics only slightly.

Attempts to isolate revertants from transformed cell populations, even using fairly powerful selective techniques, have met with only limited success—almost all such revertants are *not* resistant to *re*transformation and as such are of only limited value in assessing the mechanism of transformation. It is useful at this point to consider some of the possible mechanisms by which transformed cells can give rise to different kinds of nontransformed revertants and to list the properties of those revertants of interest.

Origins of the Revertant Phenotype: A Model

In Fig. 1 and Table 1, we describe in a very general way a scheme by which retroviral oncogenes might transform susceptible cells. Possible points at which the process of transformation can be blocked to yield nontransformed revertant cells are indicated. Although the mechanisms of cell transformation and reversion to the nontransformed phenotype are poorly understood at this time, we hope that a uniform terminology for the various kinds of revertants, coupled with diagnostic properties for various types of revertants, as shown in Table 1, will help to clarify and organize results in this area by providing a framework for the comparison of revertants isolated in different laboratories. The characteristics used here to separate the various types of revertants are strictly operational in that those revertants that behave alike are grouped together. It is anticipated that, with an increasing understanding of the pathways involved in transformation, revertants can eventually be subclassified according to the exact mechanisms responsible for reversion. It is important to note that we have not dealt here with changes in additional genes whose functions may involve the regulation of other genes or modification of their products. Should revertants resulting from changes in such regulatory genes exist, they will have properties other than those listed in Table 1, and this will result in additional complexities in the model.

In Fig. 1, the transformation of a cell is shown to result from the interaction of the products of two kinds of genes:

1. An oncogene, whose expression is essential for the process of transformation. The protein product of the oncogene, which we shall call the oncoprotein, is directly responsible for initiating the molecular changes associated with trans-

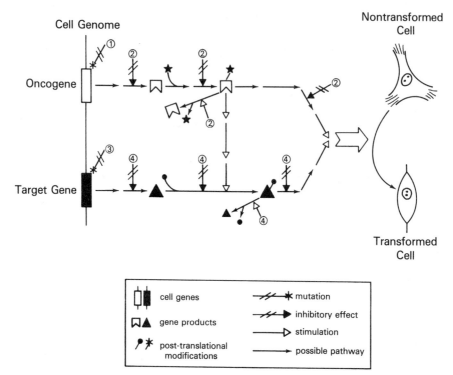

FIG. 1. A simplified scheme for transformation of a cell involving two genes; an oncogene and a target gene. Potential steps at which the revertant phenotype can be generated by inhibitory or stimulatory cellular events are indicated by numbers. Revertants generated by changes at different steps that are labeled with the same number cannot be distinguished using present methods. It is anticipated that these revertants will be further classified as more is learned about the mechanism of transformation.

formation, although the pathway(s) by which it acts may require a complex series of steps. Both "activated" proto-oncogenes and viral oncogenes introduced into the cell following transfection or infection are considered together in this model.

2. A cell-encoded "target" gene whose product or "target" molecule interacts with the oncoprotein to initiate the process of transformation. (As indicated in Fig. 1, some oncogenes may transform cells without interacting with a target molecule).

The function of either an oncogene or its target gene may be inhibited by either of two basic types of alteration, as diagrammed in Fig. 1: (a) a mutation or some other change in the structure of the gene itself (or in any of its regulatory elements), or (b) inhibition of the synthesis or function of the gene product. In total, then, there are four classes of revertants considered in this model, representing two general kinds of changes in either the oncogene or the target gene. A preliminary classification of these four classes of revertants based on their expected behavior under certain experimental conditions is given in Table 1. Two of the four rever-

TABLE 1. *Classification of revertant cells*

Property	Oncoprotein-related		Target-related	
	Oncogene-altered (Class 1)*	Oncoprotein-deficient (Class 2)*	Target Gene-altered (Class 3)*	Target-deficient (Class 4)*
Functional Oncogene	No	Yes	Yes	Yes
Active oncoprotein	No	No	Yes	Yes
Functional Target Gene	Yes	Yes	No	Yes
Active Target Molecule	Yes	Yes	No	No
Loss of all characteristics of transformation	Yes	Yes	Yes/No	Yes/No
Retransformation after infection with Ki-MuSV	Yes	No	No	No
Phenotype when Fused to Cells Transformed by:				
Original Oncogene	TF	Flat	TF	Flat
Oncogene with similar function†	TF	TF	TF	Flat
Oncogene with different function¶	TF	TF	TF	TF
Nontransformed parent	Flat	Flat	TF	TF

*Classes 1–4 correspond to numbers 1–4 in Fig. 1.
TF = transformed; Flat = nontransformed morphology.
†i.e. a structurally different oncogene that transforms via the same target molecule.
¶i.e. an oncogene which transforms via a second pathway involving a different target molecule.

tant classes are listed under a general heading called "oncoprotein-related", and the other two are listed under the heading "target-related", depending on which of the two gene products shown in Fig. 1 has been affected. (We have avoided the use of terms such as "repressor", "suppressor", and "anti-oncogene", each of which has been used already to describe resistance to transformation in other systems).

The two classes of oncoprotein-related revertants, termed "oncogene-altered" and "oncoprotein-deficient" in Table 1, correspond to the lesions numbered "1" and "2" in Fig. 1, and cells from both classes are deficient in the amount of active oncoprotein. In oncogene-altered revertants (class 1), the oncogene itself has been altered or has been lost and can no longer direct the synthesis of a sufficient amount of functional product. It is not possible to isolate an active oncogene regularly from these cells by transfection of revertant DNA or by "rescue" with a "helper" virus. A distinctive characteristic of oncogene-altered revertants is a susceptibility to *re*transformation after infection with virus particles containing the original oncogene. Also, since the transformation process is blocked at is origin in this case, all of the properties associated with transformation should disappear (unless the oncoprotein has multiple functions, and only one of them is affected). In general, oncogene-altered revertants should closely resemble the original nontransformed cells from which they were derived. Oncogene-altered revertants are the most common type of revertant isolated to date (see below). This class of revertants is not likely to yield new information regarding the mechanism of transformation.

In revertants belonging to the oncoprotein-deficient class (class 2), the transcription, translation, or function of the oncogene product is inhibited by some cellular activity. Several potential sites of inhibition for class 2 revertants are indicated in Fig. 1. Oncoprotein-deficient revertants retain an intact oncogene whose activity can be demonstrated by virus rescue or DNA-mediated transfection into susceptible cells; however, the oncoprotein is not present in an active form in these revertants. Depending on the complexity of the transformation pathway, members of the oncoprotein-deficient class of revertants could lose either one, several, or all of the characteristics associated with the transformed state. Oncoprotein-deficient revertants should be resistant to retransformation by the original oncogene with which they were transformed and possibly by other oncogenes that bear specific structural similarities to it. The nontransformed rat cells infected with Rous sarcoma virus by Dyson and co-workers (mentioned above) appear to contain a *trans*-acting inhibitor of viral transcription (15,25) and are thus analagous to class 2 revertants.

Target-related revertants (classes 3 and 4) contain oncogenes that function normally and synthesize sufficient quantities of oncoprotein to transform cells. The transformed phenotype is not expressed, however, because a cell-encoded target molecule required for transformation is deficient. Class 3, or target-gene-altered, revertants contain mutations or other changes in the target gene. Either insufficient or defective target molecules are produced, and transformation does not occur because the oncoprotein lacks its specific substrate. Target-gene-altered revertants resist retransformation following infection or transfection with the original oncogene. Unlike other revertants, however, the transformed phenotype reappears in hybrids between target-gene-altered revertants and nontransformed cells, since the latter contain a functional target gene and its product. Target-gene-altered revertants should also resist retransformation with other oncogenes that transform cells by pathways involving the same target molecule (*i.e.*, oncogenes *functionally* related to the original oncogene).

Class 4, or target-deficient, revertants possess an inhibitory activity that prevents transcription, translation, posttranslational modification, stability, or some other property of the target molecule. Again, transformation is inhibited because of the absence of functional target molecules, and the revertant should resist retransformation by the same and functionally related oncogenes. Fusion of target-deficient revertants to nontransformed parental cells should result in hybrids with a nontransformed phenotype. In those cases where the target molecule is required for cell growth, many of the alterations that would result in target-related revertants may be lethal to the cell, and the number of revertants belonging to this class may be correspondingly small. On the other hand, revertants in this class may resist retransformation by obviating the requirement for the target protein, perhaps by using substitutes or entirely different pathways to perform the same functions as the target molecule. In such cases, the phenotype of the revertant, in addition to its nontransformed characteristics, may differ in other properties from both the transformed cell line from which it was derived and the original progenitor (untransformed) cell line.

Thus, revertants from each of the four classes listed in Table 1 exhibit properties that can be defined experimentally with present techniques. Complementation studies involving two or more different revertants may also be used to define relationships, but such studies have not yet been reported. It seems that systematic comparisons of target-related revertants that have already been isolated and those that will be isolated in the future are in order.

A complete scheme describing the mechanisms of transformation and reversion should include the participation of other "cooperating" oncogenes such as "immortalization" genes described by several laboratories (48,58,70). Each of these reports demonstrated that a single retroviral oncogene such as v-*ras* is not sufficient to induce transformation in diploid embryo fibroblasts. Although the *ras* gene seems to be responsible for morphological changes in the cell, transformation is also dependent on the presence of a second gene responsible for indefinite growth of the fibroblasts. The requirement for a second or cooperating gene can be filled by viral oncogenes, such as *myc, fos, myb,* and genes from DNA transforming viruses and others. Control NIH/3T3 cells and other permanent cell lines are aleady immortalized and require only a single oncogene for the expression of the complete transformed phenotype. Examples of cooperating oncogenes are given elsewhere in this volume.

This classification of revertant cells can be applied with a few modifications to cell-fusion experiments, where inhibition of the transformed phenotype has been observed in hybrids between transformed cells and normal cells, especially human diploid fibroblasts (see above). In fusions between transformed cells and nontransformed cells of heterologous species, however, it is possible that the functions of certain enzymes or of entire pathways are different in the nontransformed partner, and the resulting hybrids, if nontransformed, may have properties similar to revertants of the target-gene-altered class.

Finally, the model that we have outlined does not take into account gene dosage effects or other quantitative aspects of transformation. Expression and loss of the transformed phenotype have been considered here to be the result of changes in individual genes and have been considered as all-or-none phenomena. In fact, however, expression of the transformed state may depend on a balance between many genes, some promoting and others inhibiting the transformed phenotype. It may be that the relative copy numbers of certain genes and the concentrations of critical proteins determine the phenotype of a cell and that transformation and reversion result from the concentrations of certain key substances within the cell. In cases such as this, the model that we have presented may be too simplified to be of value, but the basic need for organizing and testing the properties of transformed and nontransformed cells along the lines presented here remains.

Properties of Known Revertant Cell Lines

Early Studies on Revertants

Results from a number of studies on revertants isolated from *src-*, *mos-*, and *ras-* transformed cells have been reported (30,35,36,49,50,54,60–62,86,95, 101,102). Most of these experiments were carried out before the occurrence and properties of retroviral oncogenes and their transforming proteins were known, and it is usually not possible to identify the basis for the loss of a transformed pheno-type with certainty. In most cases, the revertant cells appear to lack a rescuable transforming retrovirus, and the revertants probably belong to the oncogene-altered class (class 1), as listed in Table 1. These revertants are not of great value in ana-lyzing the mechanism of transformation and shall not be considered further.

Hoffman et al. (38) used methionine-free medium to select methionine-indepen-dent clones of SV40-transformed human fibroblasts and rat tumor cells. They noted that some of the methionine-independent clones were revertants, having lost some of the properties associated with the transformed state. Viral T antigens were detected in some cases, but the class to which these revertants belong cannot be determined.

R5-5-1 Revertant

Three morphological revertants isolated from NIH/3T3 cells infected and trans-formed with Ki-MuSV were described by Morris et al. (55). After treatment with the mutagen *N'*-methyl-*N*-nitroso guanidine, the parental transformed cells were subjected to two cycles of "negative selection" with BUdR under conditions that favored the survival of nontransformed cells. From the remaining cell population, three candidate revertant clones (R1-1, R2-1, and R5-5-1) were isolated on the basis of their morphological similarity to nontransformed NIH/3T3 cells. Two of these revertants did not cause tumors in nude mice (10^6 cells injected), and the third (R5-5-1) was clearly less tumorigenic than the parental transformed cells. None of the revertants showed appreciable growth in soft agar. The integrity of the Ki-*ras* oncogene in each of the revertant lines was indicated by "rescue" of transforming K-MuSV following superinfection with a murine leukemia "helper" virus. Subsequent molecular studies (62) showed that the integrated Ki-MuSV ge-nome in each revertant was indistinguishable from that of the parental transformed cell line and that there were no apparent changes in host flanking sequences. Also, analysis with restriction endonucleases indicated that the *ras*-specific DNA in the revertants was not hypermethylated (62). As a further measure of the ability of the Ki-MuSV genome to function in the revertant cells, Ki-MuSV-specific mRNA and p21 levels were measured and found not to differ appreciably from the original transformed parental line. Data regarding the susceptibility of the revertants to re-transformation following superinfection with Ki-MuSV are difficult to interpret.

Analysis of Ki-MuSV-specific high-molecular-weight DNA in two of the revertants shortly after superinfection with high concentrations of Ki-MuSV showed the integration of additional copies of Ki-MuSV proviral DNA.

The relationships of transforming growth factors and their receptors to loss of the transformed phenotype were examined in the R5-5-1 revertant (10). There were very few EGF receptors on the surface of both the transformed and revertant cells, similar to our results with the C-11 and F-2 revertants (to be discussed later), but very little, if any, α- or β-TGF activity was detected in concentrated culture fluids from either the R5-5-1 line or the v-Ki-*ras*-transformed parental cell line, CC1. It is not possible therefore to determine whether or not these revertant cells possess fewer receptors for α-TGF than do the NIH/3T3 or CC1 cell lines or whether they secrete enough α-TGF to saturate the available binding sites (10). It is conceivable that the genetic change responsible for the revertant phenotype in R5-5-1 cells is related to the synthesis of sufficient numbers of EGF receptor. Alternatively, α-TGF production may not be required for transformation by the v-Ki-*ras* gene.

Enough data exist to place the R5-5-1 revertant into the category of target-related revertants (Table 1), largely on the basis of positive rescue experiments, demonstrating that the revertant cells contained functional v-Ki-*ras* oncogenes. Further studies, especially cell fusion experiments, are indicated in order to identify the nature of the changes in these cells. Should the phenotype of this cell result from a lack of EGF receptors, for example, this revertant would be categorized as target-deficient (class 4).

Revertants C-11 and F-2 from Ki-ras-Transformed NIH/3T3 Cells

We were originally interested in isolating revertants from Ki-MuSV-transformed cells that contained alterations in the synthesis or structure of cell-encoded target molecule(s) involved in the transformation pathway (i.e., the target-related revertants listed in Table 1). It seemed likely from previous data that if target-related revertants exist in mutagenized cultures of transformed cells, they occur much less frequently than do oncoprotein-related revertants. We therefore attempted to enrich the numbers of target-related revertants in mutagenized populations of transformed parental cells, on the one hand, and to reduce the occurrence of oncoprotein-related revertants, on the other.

The frequency of oncoprotein-related revertants was diminished by employing the doubly transformed (DT) cell line, a subline of NIH/3T3 cells that had been infected on two separate occasions with Ki-MuSV (59). Southern blot analysis indicated that there were indeed two copies of v-Ki-*ras* in the high-molecular-weight DNA extracted from DT cells (1).

Enrichment of revertants in populations of transformed DT cells treated with mutagen was achieved by selection in 1 mM ouabain (59). In searching for a suitable selective agent, we attempted to take advantage of the fact that many of the properties normally associated with transformed cells seem to involve fundamental changes in the plasma membrane. Ouabain was chosen as a potential selective agent because it is highly specific, its mechanism of action is well known, and the enzyme that it inhibits (Na^+, K^+ATPase) is located at the plasma membrane. In fact, ouabain proved to be an excellent selective agent, enriching the number of phenotypically flat (nontransformed) cells by 1,000- to 10,000-fold (1). The possible significance of the differential effect of ouabain on transformed and nontransformed cells is discussed later.

Using the DT cell line as the transformed parent together with ouabain selection, we have isolated four revertant cell lines that we believe contain active *ras* oncogenes. The frequency of occurrence of these revertants in mutagen-treated DT cells is roughly estimated to be less than one in 10^7. Some of the characteristics of the two revertants (C-11 and F-2) that we have studied in more detail are compared with those of the original nontransformed NIH/3T3 cell line and the transformed parent line DT and are summarized in Table 2. The biological and molecular properties of the revertant cells can be classified into three general categories: (a) those associated with the original NIH/3T3 cell line; (b) those associated with the continued expression of the *ras* oncogene; and (c) those that appear to be unique to the revertant cells themselves.

A number of the biological properties that are characteristic of the DT cell appear to be altered or missing in the revertants. Thus, revertant cells exhibit low saturation densities when grown as monolayers, do not form multilayers, and do not multiply in agar suspension cultures (59). Moreover, when inoculated into nude mice, the C-11 and F-2 revertant cell lines show little or no tumorigenicity. Thus, the C-11 and F-2 revertants contain elevated levels of the transforming protein p21 but have lost at least some of the properties associated with transformation by the *ras* gene.

As described in Table 1 and Fig. 1, the nature of the genetic change responsible for reversion of a cell to the nontransformed phenotype can be deduced from the behavior of the cell under certain experimental conditions. As indicated by the Southern blot technique, the C-11 and F-2 revertant cell lines each retain the same two copies of the v-Ki-*ras* gene as does the original DT line from which they were derived (1), although small changes such as point mutations in the DNA sequence are not detectable with this method. The quantity of the oncoprotein, (i.e., the *ras* gene product p21) is greater than that in NIH/3T3 cells but somewhat less than that seen in DT cells (1).

In addition to the molecular studies described above, we have also determined the ability of the v-Ki-*ras* genomes present in the C-11 and F-2 revertants to initiate and maintain the transformed phenotype when introduced into nontransformed cells, including the original NIH/3T3 cell line. The C-11 and F-2 cells were superinfected with ecotropic or amphotropic MuLV, and the proportion of cells containing a rescuable transforming virus was determined by infectious center assay. Essentially 100% of the C-11 and F-2 revertant cells were capable of producing transforming virus in this assay (1). Furthermore, transforming activity in preparations of high-molecular-weight DNA extracted from revertant cells could be demonstrated directly in transfection experiments. On the basis of these results, the C-11 and F-2 revertants do not appear to belong to the oncogene-altered class of revertants described in Table 1.

Culture fluids from revertants C-11 and F-2 were also examined for evidence of low-molecular-weight transforming growth factors (TGFs) (75). TGFs are a group of polypeptide growth-stimulating factors found in the culture fluids of cells transformed by a number of retroviral oncogenes, including *ras* [see Salomon and Perroteau (74) for review]. Concentrated culture fluids from both the DT cell line and the C-11 and F-2 revertants were capable of stimulating NRK cells to grow in agar suspension cultures, whereas control NIH/3T3 cell fluids were negative (75). Furthermore, studies with ^{125}I-labeled EGF showed that the revertant cells, like the parental DT cells, contain very few unoccupied EGF receptor sites, another indication that revertant cells secrete α-TGF into the culture fluids (75). A lack of receptor sites resulting from some other change cannot be excluded. In another experiment, addition of active α-TGF preparations to the revertant cells did not result in agar growth or in morphological changes, as it did in control (nontransformed) cells. These studies with tumor growth factors indicate that the C-11 and F-2 revertants, unlike the R5-5-1 revertant described above, are able to direct the synthesis of α-TGF but appear to be resistant to its effects, presumably because of some alteration at a point in the transformation pathway distal to the interaction of TGF with its receptor. The ability of these revertant cells to multiply in medium with low serum (Table 2) may be the result of TGF production.

From the data presented so far, revertants C-11 and F-2 appear to contain a functioning *ras* gene and therefore belong to the target-related group of revertants described in Table 1. Although the exact role of TGF in cell transformation by the *ras* oncogene is not yet clear, its synthesis and the other properties mentioned

TABLE 2. *Molecular and biological properties of NIH/3T3, DT, and revertants C-11 and F-2*

Property	Cell line			
	NIH/3T3	DT	C-11	F-2
Morphology	Flat	TF	Flat	Flat
Colony-forming activity (%)				
10% serum	43	74	41	48
1% serum	1.7	16	14	13
soft agar	<0.01	22	<0.03	<0.01
Ouabain sensitivity	Low	High	Low	Low
Tumorigenicity (nude mice)	−	+	−	−
Tropomyosin synthesis	+	−	+	+
Growth factor production	−	+	+	+
v-Ki-*ras* sequences	−	+	+	+
Elevated levels of p21	−	+	+	+
Rescuable Ki-MuSV	−	+	+	+
Chromosomes	61	60	93	88
Relative cell volume	1.00	1.04	1.64	1.33

above indicate that the C-11 and F-2 revertants may belong to the target-deficient class of revertants described in Table 1.

Another critical diagnostic property of revertants that can be used to separate oncogene-deficient from target-related revertants is the ability to resist retransformation when challenged with additional copies of the original transforming oncogene, in this case, v-Ki-*ras*, or with other oncogenes that may be either structurally or functionally related to *ras*. The susceptibility of the C-11 and F-2 revertant cell lines to retransformation by v-Ki-*ras* as well as by other oncogenes was assessed by two different techniques: (a) analysis of hybrid cells resulting from the fusion of revertants to NIH/3T3 cell lines transformed by a variety of retroviral oncogenes, by papovaviruses, or by chemical carcinogens; or (b) direct superinfection of the revertant cells by transforming retroviruses or by transfection with appropriate DNAs.

Cell fusions, following treatment with polyethylene glycol, were carried out with revertant, control, and transformed cell lines containing appropriate selectable markers. We usually employed the system of Ozer and Jha (64), fusing doubly marked (thioguanine-resistant and ouabain-resistant) derivatives of the revertant cell line to wild-type transformed cells and selecting the resulting hybrids in medium containing HAT and ouabain. Hybridizations were carried out at cell densities that precluded fusion of more than two cells per hybrid to minimize gene dosage effects. Hybrid cells were scored for the presence or absence of the transformed phenotype based on their appearance in monolayer cultures or their growth in agar suspension cultures (59).

Important control experiments indicated, first, that the transformed phenotype was dominant in hybrids between control NIH/3T3 cells and all transformed cells tested. Therefore transformation by these oncogenes was probably not the result of an *absence* of genetic material, as described for Wilm's tumor and other heritable neoplasms. This control indicated that there was no expression of the transformed phenotype in hybrids between either of the revertants and untransformed NIH/3T3 cells. The C-11 and F-2 revertants therefore do not appear to be target-gene-altered (class 3, as described in Table 1).

The expression of the revertant phenotype in hybrids between either the C-11 or F-2 cell line and a number of transformed cells was assessed by a series of cell fusion experiments (59). Usually, two or more different cell lines transformed by the same oncogene were fused to each of the revertants. Based on the behavior of various cell lines in these experiments and taking into account the results of fusion of the same transformed cell lines to control NIH/3T3 cells, it is possible to divide retroviral oncogenes and other transforming agents into two groups: those whose expression is dominant over the revertant phenotype, and those whose expression is not dominant. In Table 3, the results of a large number of cell fusion experiments are summarized.

The three oncogenes that are inhibited by revertants C-11 and F-2 (*ras, src,* and *fes*) encode products that are not closely related in structure to one another. This suggests that the resistance pattern seen in Table 3 is a result of a block in some

TABLE 3. *Functional classification of transforming agents based on cell hybridization experiments*

Repressed by C-11 and F-2	Not repressed
Ki-*ras*	*mos*
Ha-*ras*	*sis*
N-*ras*	*fms*
c-Ha-*ras* 1 (human)	Polyoma
bas	SV40
fes	Chemically transformed (10 lines)
src	

part of a converging functional pathway by which *ras, src,* and *fes* induce cell transformation. Available results provide only limited information regarding the nature of transformation pathways at this time. Nevertheless, the C-11 and F-2 revertants may be able to discriminate among oncogenes at a functional rather than structural level, a potentially valuable clue into the mechanism of transformation by different oncogenes. Superinfection of the C-11 and F-2 lines with different transforming viruses indicated the same resistance pattern as did the fusion experiments (1).

On the basis of the above data, it seems most likely that the C-11 and F-2 are target-related revertants of the target-deficient class. The fact that the revertant cell lines contain a higher number of chromosomes than do the transformed DT cells from which they were derived may indicate that quantitative phenomena (gene dosage effects) are responsible for resistance to retransformation. This possibility is under study.

Revertants C-11 and F-2 have also been examined by two-dimensional gel electrophoresis in an attempt to find individual proteins that vary with the *ras*-transformed phenotype. In a study by Cooper et al. (17), NIH/3T3, DT, and C-11 and F-2 cells were labeled with [^{3}H]leucine and analyzed on two-dimensional polyacrylamide gels. The amounts of only two proteins, both forms of nonmuscle tropomyosin, were consistently altered (reduced) in *ras*-transformed cells and restored to control levels in the revertant cell lines. In fact, cells transformed by several retroviral oncogenes (but not by polyoma or SV40) showed changes in tropomyosin synthesis.

The role of tropomyosin in the transformation process is currently under investigation, but it is interesting to note that the removal of tropomyosin from cell membrane preparations is associated with a marked increase in the sensitivity of the accompanying Na^+, K^+-ATPase to inactivation by ouabain. Conversely, addition of tropomysin to such free-membrane preparations restores the ouabain resistance of the Na^+,K^+ ATPase (51). Thus, the ouabain sensitivity of *ras*-transformed NIH/3T3 cells noted previously (1,59) and the disappearance of tropomyosin from the membranes of *ras*-transformed cells (17) both may be manifestations of the same (still unknown) basic property of transformed cells. It will be interesting to see if tropomyosin synthesis in the revertant cells differs in any way from that in the parental NIH/3T3 cells.

FUTURE STUDIES

The mechanisms underlying the sensitivity of transformed cells to ouabain are currently under investigation. Ki-*ras*-transformed human HOS cells are also much more sensitive to ouabain than are their nontransformed counterparts. This effect is independent of the 1,000-fold increase in sensitivity to ouabain exhibited by the human control cells. In both human and mouse cells, the effects of ouabain appear to be dependent on the pH of the culture medium, toxicity being more evident at alkaline pH (L. Benade, *unpublished data*). Since ouabain is a specific inhibitor of Na^+,K^+ ATPase, we are currently investigating possible differences in monovalent cation transport in normal, *ras*-transformed, and revertant cells.

Another approach to understanding the mechanism of transformation using revertants is concerned with identifying the genetic change responsible for the revertant phenotype using DNA-mediated transfection techniques. High-molecular-weight DNA has been extracted from revertant cells and used to cotransfect the DT cell line together with the plasmid pSV2 *neo*. A small number of cells that appear to express the nontransformed phenotype have been recovered in these experiments, but it has not yet been confirmed that they contain the sequences responsible for the revertant phenotype. These and other transfection studies are now in progress. Additional experiments using a rat fibroblast cell line infected with two copies of the v-Ki-*ras* gene as a recipient for transfection experiments and DNA extracted from the revertants have been initiated.

Studies with revertants specifically resistant to individual oncogenes have given us at least three possible approaches to characterize the mechanism of action of the *ras* retroviral oncogene: (a) a study of ion transport systems to discover the basis of the sensitivity of *ras*-transformed cells to ouabain; (b) a study of tropomyosin synthesis is transformed and nontransformed cells; and (c) a molecular approach designed to identify the gene responsible for the revertant phenotype. The isolation of additional target-related revertants from other oncogenes will also help in defining the mechanisms by which transformation can be inhibited and thus in learning more about the nature of the pathways themselves.

ACKNOWLEDGMENTS

We wish to thank Brenda Wallace-Jones and Bud Strong for their expert technical assistance with those studies reported from our laboratory. Drs. Pierosandro Tagliaferri and David Salomon, of NIH, and Dr. Leonard Benade, American Type Culture Collection, Kensington, Maryland, were most helpful in the preparation of the manuscript.

REFERENCES

1. Bassin, R.H., Noda, M., Scolnick, E.M., and Selinger, Z.S. (1984): Study of possible relationships among retroviral oncogenes using flat revertants isolated from Kirsten sarcoma virus-transformed cells. In: *Cancer Cells, Vol. 2: Oncogenes and Viral Genes*, edited by G.F. Vande Woude, A.J. Levine, W.I. Topp, and J.D. Watson, pp. 463–471. Cold Spring Harbor Laboratory Press. Cold Spring Harbor, New York.
2. Beckner, S.K., Hattori, S., and Shih, T.Y. (1985): The *ras* oncogene product p21 is not a regulatory component of adenylate cyclase. *Nature*, 317:71–72.
3. Benedict, W.F., Weissman, B.E., Mark, C., and Stanbridge, E.J. (1984): Tumorigenicity of human HT1080 fibrosarcoma × normal fibroblast hybrids: Chromosome dosage dependency. *Cancer Res.*, 44:3471–3479.
4. Bishop, J.M. (1983): Cellular oncogenes and retroviruses. *Ann. Rev. Biochem.*, 52:301–354.
5. Bishop, J.M. (1985): Viral oncogenes. *Cell*, 42:23–38.
6. Bishop, J.M., and Varmus, H.E. (1982): Functions and origins of retroviral transforming genes. In: *Molecular Biology of Tumor Viruses. Part III. RNA Tumor Viruses.*, edited by R. Weiss, N. Teich, H. Varmus, and J. Coffin, pp. 999–1108. Cold Spring Harbor Press, Cold Spring Harbor, New York.
7. Bouck, N., and di Mayorca, G. (1976): Somatic mutation as the basis for malignant transformation of BHK cells by chemical carcinogens. *Nature*, 264:722–727.
8. Bouck, N., and di Mayorca, G. (1982): Chemical carcinogens transform BHK cells by inducing a recessive mutation. *Mol. Cell. Biol.*, 2:97–105.
9. Broek, D., Samiy, N., Fasano, O., Fujiyama, A., Tamanoi, F., Northrup, J., and Wigler, M. (1985): Differential activation of yeast adenylate cyclase by wild-type and mutant *RAS* proteins. *Cell*, 41:763–769.
10. Brown, K.D., Blakeley, D.M., Roberts, P., and Avery, R.J. (1985): Loss of epidermal growth factor receptors and release of transforming growth factors do not correlate with sarcoma virus transformation in clonally related NIH/3T3-derived cell lines. *Biochem. J.*, 229:119–125.
11. Campisi, J., Gray, H.E., Pardee, A.B., Dean, M., and Sonenshein, G.E. (1984): Cell-cycle control of c-*myc* but not c-*ras* expression is lost following chemical transformation. *Cell*, 36:241–247.
12. Cavenee, W.K., Hansen, M.F., Nordenskjold, M., Kock, E., Maumenee, I., Squire, J.A., Phillips, R.A., and Gallie, B.L. (1985): Genetic origin of mutations predisposing to retinoblastoma. *Science*, 228:501–503.
13. Chang, E.H., Furth, M.E., Scolnick, E.M., and Lowy, D.R. (1982): Tumourigenic transformation of mammalian cells induced by a normal human gene homologous to the oncogene of Harvey murine sarcoma virus. *Nature*, 297:479–483.
14. Chang, E.H., Gonda, M.A., Ellis, R.W., Scolnick, E.M., and Lowy, D.R. (1982): Human genome contains four genes homologous to transforming genes of Harvey and Kirsten murine sarcoma viruses. *Proc. Natl. Acad. Sci. U.S.A.*, 79:4848–4852.
15. Chiswell, D.J., Enrietto, P.J., Evans, S., Quade, K., and Wyke, J.A. (1982): Molecular mechanisms involved in morphological variation of avian sarcoma virus-infected rat cells. *Virology*, 116:428–440.
16. Collett, M.S., and Erikson, R.L. (1978): Protein kinase activity associated with the avian sarcoma virus *src* gene product. *Proc. Natl. Acad. Sci. U.S.A.*, 75:2021–2024.
17. Cooper, H.L., Feuerstein, N., Noda, M., and Bassin, R.H. (1985): Suppression of tropomyosin synthesis, a common biochemical feature of oncogenesis by structurally diverse retroviral oncogenes. *Mol. Cell. Biol.*, 5:952–983.
18. Craig, R.W., and Sager, R. (1985): Suppression of tumorigenicity in hybrids of normal and oncogene-transformed CHEF cells. *Proc. Natl. Acad. Sci. U.S.A.*, 82:2062–2066.
19. De Feo-Jones, D., Scolnick, E.M., Koller, R., and Dhar, R. (1983): *ras*-Related sequences identified and isolated from *Saccharomyces cerevesiae*. *Nature*, 306:707–709.
20. De Feo-Jones, D., Tatchell, K., Robinson, L.C., Sigal, I.S., Vass, W.C., Lowy, D.R., and Scolnick, E.M. (1985): Mammalian and yeast *ras* gene products: Biological function in their heterologous systems. *Science*, 228:179–184.
21. Der, C.J., Krontiris, T.G., and Cooper, G.M. (1982): Transforming genes of human bladder and lung carcinoma cell lines are homologous to the *ras* genes of Harvey and Kirsten sarcoma viruses. *Proc. Natl. Acad. Sci. U.S.A.*, 79:3637–3640.

22. Doolittle, R.F., Hunkapiller, M.W., Hood, L.E., DeVare, S.G., Robbins, K.C., Aaronson, S.A., and Antoniades, H.N. (1983): Simian sarcoma virus *onc*-gene v-*sis* is derived from the gene (or genes) encoding a platelet-derived growth factor. *Science,* 221:275–276.

23. Downward, J., Yarden, B., Mayes, B., Scrace, G., Totley, N., Stockwell, P., Ulrich, A., Schlessinger, J., and Waterfield, M.D. (1984): Close similarity of epidermal growth factor receptor and v-*erb*-B oncogene protein sequences. *Nature,* 307:521–527.

24. Duesberg, P.H. (1985): Activated proto-*onc*-genes: Sufficient or necessary for cancer? *Science,* 228:669–677.

25. Dyson, P.J., Cook, P.R., Searle, S., and Wyke, J.A. (1985): The chromatin structure of Rous sarcoma proviruses is changed by factors that act in *trans* in cell hybrids. *EMBO J.,* 4:413–420.

26. Dyson, P.J., Quade, K., and Wyke, J.A. (1982): Molecular mechanisms involved in morphological variation of avian sarcoma virus-infected rat cells. *Virology,* 116:428–440.

27. Dyson, P.J., Quade, K., and Wyke, J.A. (1982): Expression of the ASV *src* gene in hybrids between normal and virally transformed cells: Specific suppression occurs in some hybrids but not others. *Cell,* 30:491–498.

28. Fernandez-Pol, J.A., Hamilton, P.D., and Klos, J.D. (1982): Correlation between the loss of the transformed phenotype and an increase in superoxide dismutase activity in a revertant subclone of sarcoma virus-infected mammalian cells. *Cancer Res.,* 42:609–617.

29. Fischinger, P.J., Blevins, C.S., Frankel, A.E., Tuttle-Fuller, N., Haapala, D.K., Nomura, S., and Robey, W.G. (1981): Biological, immunological, and molecular properties of revertants of cat cells transformed by murine sarcoma virus. *Cancer Res.,* 41:958–965.

30. Fischinger, P.J., Nomura, S., Peebles, P.T., Haapala, D.K., and Bassin, R.H. (1972): Reversion of murine sarcomavirus-transformed mouse cells: Variants without a rescuable sarcoma virus. *Science,* 176:1033–1035.

31. Goldfarb, M., Shimizu, K., Perucho, M., and Wigler, M. (1982): Isolation and preliminary characterization of a human transforming gene from T24 bladder carcinoma cells. *Nature,* 296:404–409.

32. Goyette, M., Petropoulos, C.J., Shank, P.R., and Fausto, N. (1983): Expression of a cellular oncogene during liver regeneration. *Science,* 219:510–512.

33. Goyette, M., Petropoulos, C.J., Shank, P.R., and Fausto, N. (1984): Regulated transcription of ci-Ki-*ras* and c-*myc* during compensatory growth of rat liver. *Mol. Cell Biol.,* 4:1493–1498.

34. Green, A.R., and Wyke, J.A. (1985): Anti-oncogenes. A subset of regulatory genes involved in carcinogenesis? *Lancet,* No. 8543, 2:475–477.

35. Greenberger, J.S., Anderson, G.R., and Aaronson, S.A. (1974): Transformation-defective virus mutants in a class of morphological revertants of sarcoma virus-transformed nonproducer cells. *Cell,* 2:279–286.

36. Greenberger, J.S., Bensinger, W.I., and Aaronson, S.A. (1976): Selective techniques for the isolation of morphological revertants of sarcoma virus-transformed cells. In: *Methods in Cell Biology,* edited by D.M. Prescott, pp. 238–249. Academic Press, New York.

37. Harris, H., Miller, O.J., Klein, G., Worst, P., and Tachibana, T. (1969): Suppression of malignancy by cell fusion. *Nature,* 223:363–367.

38. Hoffman, R.M., Jacobsen, S.J., and Erbe, R.W. (1979): Reversion to methionine independence in simian virus 40-transformed human and malignant rat fibroblasts is associated with altered ploidy and altered properties of transformation. *Proc. Natl. Acad. Sci. U.S.A.,* 76:1313–1317.

39. Hunter, T., and Cooper, J.A. (1983): Role of tyrosine phosphorylation in malignant transformation by viruses and in cellular growth control. *Proc. Nucl. Acid Res. Mol. Biol.,* 29:221–232.

40. Jurnak, F. (1985): Structure of the GDP domain of EF-Tu and location of the amino acids homologous to *ras* oncogene proteins. *Science,* 230:32–36.

41. Kataoka, T., Powers, S., Cameron, S., Fasano, O., Goldfarb, M., Broach, J., and Wigler, M. (1985): Functional homology of mammalian and yeast *ras* genes. *Cell,* 40:19–26.

42. Kataoka, T., Powers, S., McGill, C., Fasano, O., Strathern, J., Broach, J., and Wigler, M. (1984): Genetic analysis of yeast *RAS1* and *RAS2* genes. *Cell,* 37:437–445.

43. Kelly, K., Cochran, B.H., Stiles, C.D., and Leder, P. (1983): Cell-specific regulation of the c-*myc* gene by lymphocyte mitogens and platelet-derived growth factor. *Cell,* 35:603–610.

44. Klein, G., and Klein, E. (1985): Evolution of tumours and the impact of molecular oncology. *Nature,* 315:190–195.

45. Klinger, H.P., and Shows, T.B. (1983): Suppression of tumorigenicity in somatic cell hybrids. II. Human chromosomes implicated as suppressors of tumorigenicity in hybrids with Chinese hamster ovary cells. *J. Natl. Cancer Inst.,* 71:559–569.

46. Knudson, A.G. (1985): Hereditary cancer, oncogenes, and anti-oncogenes. *Cancer Res.,* 45:1437–1443.
47. Kruijer, W., Cooper, J.A., Hunter, T., and Verma, I.M. (1984): Platelet-derived growth factor induces rapid but transient expression of the c-*fos* gene and protein. *Nature,* 312:711–716.
48. Land, H., Parada, L.F., and Weinberg, R.A. (1983): Tumorigenic conversion of primary embryo fibroblasts requires at least two cooperating oncogenes. *Nature,* 304:596–602.
49. Lau, A.F., Krzyzek, R.A., Brugge, J.S., Erikson, R.L., Schollmeyer, J., and Faras, A.J. (1979): Morphological revertants of an avian sarcoma virus-transformed mammalian cell line exhibit tumorigenicity and contain pp60^{src}. *Proc. Nat. Acad. Sci. U.S.A.,* 76:3904–3908.
50. Lau, A.F., Krzyzek, R.A., and Faras, A.J. (1981): Loss of tumorigenicity correlates with a reduction in pp60^{src} kinase activity in a revertant subclone of avian sarcoma virus-infected field vole cells. *Cell,* 23:815–823.
51. Lelievre, L.G., Potter, J.D., Piascik, M., Wallick, E.T., Schwartz, A., Charlemagne, D., and Geny, B. (1985): Specific involvement of calmodulin and non-specific effect of tropomyosin in the sensitivity to ouabain of Na$^+$,K$^+$ATPase in murine glasmacytoma cells. *Eur. J. Biochem.,* 148:13–19.
52. Liotta, L.A. (1985): Mechanisms of cancer invasion and metastases. In: *Progress in Oncology, Vol. 1,* edited by V.T. De Vita, A. Hellman, and S. Rosenberg, pp. 28–41. J.B. Lippincott, Philadelphia.
53. Marshall, C. (1985): Human oncogenes. In: *Molecular Biology of Tumor Viruses, Vol. II: RNA Tumor Viruses,* edited by R. Weiss N. Teich, H. Varmus, and J. Coffin, 2nd ed., pp. 487–558. Cold Spring Harbor Press, Cold Spring Harbor, New York.
54. Mathey-Prevot, B., Shibuya, M., Samarut, J., and Hanafusa, H. (1984): Revertants and partial transformants of rat fibroblasts infected with Fujinami sarcoma virus. *J. Virol.,* 50:325–334.
55. Morris, A., Clegg, C., Jones, J., Rodgers, B., and Avery, R.J. (1980): The isolation and characterization of a clonally related series of murine retrovirus-infected mouse cells. *J. Genet. Virol.,* 49:105–113.
56. Muller, R., and Verma, I.M., (1984): Expression of cellular oncogenes. *Curr. Top. Microbiol. Immunol.,* 112:73–146.
57. Murphree, A.L., and Benedict, W.F. (1984): Retinoblastoma: Clues to human oncogenesis. *Science,* 223:1028–1033.
58. Newbold, R.F., and Overell, R.W. (1983): Fibroblast immortality is a prerequisite for transformation by EJ c-Ha-*ras* oncogene. *Nature,* 304:648–651.
59. Noda, M., Selinger, Z., Scolnick, E., and Bassin, R.H. (1983): Flat revertants.isolated from Kirsten sarcoma virus-transformed cells are resistant to the action of specific oncogenes. *Proc. Natl. Acad. Sci. U.S.A.,* 80:5602–5606.
60. Nomura, S., Fischinger, P.J., Mattern, C.F.T., Gerwin, B.I., and Dunn, K.J. (1973): Revertants of mouse cells transformed by murine sarcoma virus. II. Flat revertants induced by fluorodeoxyuridine and colcemid. *Virology,* 56:152–163.
61. Nomura, S., Fischinger, P.J., Mattern, C.F.T., Peebles, P.T., Bassin, R.H., and Friedman, G.P. (1972): Revertants of mouse cells transformed by murine sarcoma virus. I. Characterization of flat and transformed sublines without a rescuable murine sarcoma virus. *Virology,* 50:51–64.
62. Norton, J.D., Cook, F., Roberts, P.C., Clewley, J.P., and Avery, R.J. (1984): Expression of Kirsten murine sarcoma virus in transformed, nonproducer, and revertant NIH/3T3 cells: Evidence for cell-mediated resistance to a viral oncogene in phenotypic reversion. *J. Virol.,* 50:439–444.
63. Oppermann, H., Levinson, A.D., and Varmus, H.E. (1981): The structure and protein kinase activity of proteins encoded by nonconditional mutants and back mutants in the *src* gene of avian sarcoma virus. *Virology,* 108:47–70.
64. Ozer, H.L., and Jha, K.K. (1977): Malignancy and transformation: Expression in somatic cell hybrids and variants. *Adv. Cancer Res.,* 25:53–93.
65. Parada, L., Tabin, C., Shih, C., and Weinberg, R. (1982): Human EJ bladder carcinoma oncogene is a homologue of Harvey sarcoma virus *ras* gene. *Nature,* 297:474–478.
66. Peehl, D.M., and Stanbridge, E.J. (1981): Characterization of human keratinocyte × HeLa somatic cell hybrids. *Int. J. Cancer,* 27:625–635.
67. Perotti, N., Taylor, S.I., Richert, N.D., Rapp, U.R., Pastan, I.H., and Roth, J. (1985): Immunoprecipitation of insulin receptors from cultured human lymphocytes (IM-9 cells) by antibodies to pp60^{src}. *Science,* 227:761–763.

126 ONCOGENE INHIBITION BY CELLULAR GENES

68. Powers, S., Katoaka, T., Fasano, O., Goldfarb, M., Strathern, J., Broach, J., and Wigler, M. (1984): Genes in *S. cerevesiae* encoding proteins with domains homologous to the mammalian *ras* proteins. *Cell,* 36:607–612.
69. Racker, E., Resnick, R.J., and Feldman, R. (1985): Glycolysis and methylaminoisobutyrate uptake in rat-1 cells transfected with *ras* or *myc* oncogenes. *Proc. Natl. Acad. Sci. U.S.A.,* 82:3535–3538.
70. Ruley, H.E. (1983): Adenovirus early-region 1A enables viral and cellular transforming genes to transform primary cells in culture. *Nature,* 304:602–606.
71. Sager, R. (1984): Resistance of human cells to oncogenic transformation. In: *Cancer Cells, Vol. 2: Oncogenes and Viral Genes,* edited by G.F. Vande Woude, A.J. Levine, W.I. Topp, and J.D. Watson, pp. 487–493. Cold Spring Harbor Laboratory Press, Cold Spring Harbor, New York.
72. Sager, R. (1985): Genetic suppression of tumor formation. *Adv. Cancer Res.,* 44:43–68.
73. Sager, R., and Craig, R.W. (1985): Anti-oncogenes and the suppression of tumor formation. In: *Cancer Cells, Vol. 3: Growth Factors and Transformation,* edited by J. Feramisco, B. Ozanne, and C. Stiles, pp. 95–100. Cold Spring Harbor Laboratory Press, Cold Spring Harbor, New York.
74. Salomon, D.S., and Perroteau, I. (1986): Growth factors in cancer and their relationship to oncogenes. *Cancer Invest.,* 4(1):43–60.
75. Salomon, D.S., Zwiebel, J.S., Noda, M., and Bassin, R.H. (1984): Flat revertants derived from Kirsten murine sarcoma virus-transformed cells produce transforming growth factors. *J. Cell. Physiol.,* 121:22–30.
76. Santos, E., Tronick, S.R., Aaronson, S.A., Pulciani, S., and Barbacid, M. (1982): T24 human bladder carcinoma oncogene is an activated form of the normal human homologue of BALB- and Harvey-MSV-transforming genes. *Nature,* 298:343–347.
77. Schafer, R., Doehmer, J., Druge, P.M., Rademacher, I., and Willecke, K. (1981): Genetic analysis of transformed and malignant phenotypes in somatic cell hybrids between tumorigenetic Chinese hamster cells and diploid mouse fibroblasts. *Cancer Res.,* 41:1214–1221.
78. Schafer, R., Hoffman, H., and Willecke, K. (1983): Suppression of tumorigenicity in hybrids of tumorigenic Chinese hamster cells and diploid mouse fibroblasts: Dependence on the presence of at least three different mouse chromosomes and independence of hamster genome dosage. *Cancer Res.,* 43:2240–2246.
79. Sherr, C., Rettenmier, C.W., Sacca, R., Roussel, M., Look, A.T., and Stanley, E.R. (1985): The *fms* proto-oncogene product is related to the receptor for the mononuclear phagocyte growth factor. *Cell,* 41:665–676.
80. Shih, T.Y., Papageorge, A.G., Stokes, P.E., Weeks, M.O., and Scolnick, E.M. (1980): Guanine nucleotide-binding and autophosphorylating activities associated with the p21^{src} protein of Harvey murine sarcoma virus. *Nature,* 287:686–691.
81. Shih, T.Y., and Weeks, M.O. (1984): Oncogenes and cancer: The p21 *ras* genes. *Cancer Invest.,* 2:109–123.
82. Slamon, D.J., and Cline, M.J. (1984): Expression of cellular oncogenes during embryonic and fetal development of the mouse. *Proc. Natl. Acad. Sci. U.S.A.,* 81:7141–7145.
83. Slamon, D.J., deKernion, J.B., Verma, I.M., and Cline, M.J. (1984): Expression of cellular oncogenes in human malignancies. *Science,* 224:256–262.
84. Stanbridge, E.J. (1976): Suppression of malignancy in human cells. *Nature,* 260:17–20.
85. Stanbridge, E.J., Der, C.J., Doersen, C.-J., Nishimi, R.Y., Peehl, D.M., Weissman, B.E., and Wilkinson, J.E. (1982): Human cell hybrids: Analysis of transformation and tumorigienicity. *Science,* 215:252–259.
86. Stanbridge, E.J., Flandermeyer, R.R., Daniels, D.W., and Nelson-Rees, W.A. (1981): Specific chromosome loss associated with the expression of tumorigenicity in human cell hybrids. *Somatic Cell Genet.,* 7:699–712.
87. Stephenson, J.R., Reynolds, R.K., and Aaronson, S.A. (1973): Characterization of morphological revertants of murine and avian sarcoma virus-transformed cells. *J. Virol.,* 11:218–222.
88. Stoler, A., and Bouck, N. (1985): Identification of a single chromosome in the normal human genome essential for suppression of hamster cell transformation. *Proc. Natl. Acad. Sci. U.S.A.,* 82:570–574.
89. Sukumar, S., Notario, V., Martin-Zanca, D., and Barbacid, M. (1983): Induction of mammary carcinomas in rats by nitroso-methylurea involves malignant activation of H.-*ras*-1 locus by single-point mutations. *Nature,* 306:658–661.

90. Sweet, R.W., Yokoyama, S., Kamata, T., Feramisco, J.R., Rosenberg, M., and Gross, M. (1984). The product of *ras* is a GTPase and the T24 oncogenic mutant is deficient is this activity. *Nature,* 311:273–275.

91. Tatchell, K., Chaleff, D.T., DeFeo-Jones, D., and Scolnick, E.M. (1984): Requirement of either of a pair of *ras*-related genes of *Saccharomyces cerevesiae* for spore viability. *Nature,* 309:523–527.

92. Toda, T., Uno, I., Ishikawa, T., Powers, S., Kataoka, T., Broek, D., Broach, J., Cameron, S., Matsumoto, K., and Wigler, M. (1985): In yeast, *RAS* proteins are controlling elements of adenylate cyclase. *Cell,* 40:27–36.

93. Ullrich, A., Bell, J.R., Chen, E.Y., Herrera, R., Petruzzelli, L.M., Dull, T.J., Gray, A., Coussens, L., Liao, Y.-C., Tsubokawa, M., Mason, A., Seeburg, P.H., Grunfeld, C., Rosen, O.M., and Ramachandran, J. (1985): Human insulin receptor and its relationship to the tyrosine kinase family of oncogenes. *Nature,* 313:756–761.

94. Ullrich, A., Coussens, L., Hayflick, J.S., Dull, T.J., Gray, A., Tam, A.W., Lee, J., Yarden, Y., Libermann, T.A., Schlessinger, J., Downward, J., Mayes, E.L.V., Whittle, N., Waterfield, M.D., and Seeburg, P.H. (1984): Human epidermal growth factor receptor cDNA sequence and aberrant expression of the amplified gene in A 431 epidermoid carcinoma cells. *Nature,* 309:418–425.

95. Varmus, H.E., Quintrell, N., Ortiz, S., (1981): Retroviruses as mutagens: Insertion and excision of a nontransforming provirus alter expression of a resident transforming provirus. *Cell,* 25:23–36.

96. Waterfield, M.D., Scrace, G.T., Whittle, N., Stroobant, P., Johnson, A., Wasteson, A., Westermark, B., Heldin, C.-H., Huang, J.S., and Deuel, T. (1983): Platelet-derived growth factor is structurally related to the putative transforming protein p28^{sis} of simian sarcoma virus. *Nature,* 304:35–38.

97. Weinstein, I.B., Horowitz, A.D., Fisher, P., Ivanovic, V., Gattoni-Celli, S., and Kirshmeier, P. (1982): Mechanisms of multistage carcinogenesis and their relevance to tumor cell heterogeneity. In: *Tumor Cell Heterogeneity, Origins and Implications,* edited by A.H. Owens, D.S. Coffey, and S.B. Baylin, pp. 261–283. Academic Press, New York.

98. Weiss, R., Teich, N., Varmus, H., and Coffin, J. (1982): *Molecular Biology of Tumor Viruses. Vol. 2: RNA Tumor Viruses, 2nd ed. Cold Spring Harbor Laboratory Press,* Cold Spring Harbor, New York.

99. Westin, E.H., Wong-Staal, F., Gelmann, E.P., Dalla Favera, R., Papas, T.S., Lautenberger, J.A., Eva, A., Reddy, E.P., Tronick, S.R., Aaronson, S.A., and Gallo, R.C. (1982): Expression of cellular homologues of retroviral *onc* genes in human hematopoietic cells. *Proc. Natl. Acad. Sci. U.S.A.,* 79:2490–2494.

100. Willingham, M.C., Pastan, I., Shih, T.Y., and Scolnick, E.M. (1980): Localization of the *src* gene product of the Harvey strain of murine sarcoma virus to the plasma membrane of transformed cells by electron microscopic immunocytochemistry. *Cell,* 19:1005–1014.

101. Wyke, J.A., Beamand, J.A., and Varmus, H.E. (1980): Factors affecting phenotypic reversion of rat cells transformed by avian sarcoma virus. *Cold Spring Harbor Symp. Quant. Biol.,* 14:1065–1075.

102. Wyke, J.A., and Quade, K. (1980): Infection of rat cells by avian sarcoma virus: Factors affecting transformation and subsequent reversion. *Virology,* 106:217–233.

103. Yaswen, P., Goyette, M., Shank, P.R., and Fausto, N. (1985): Expression of c-Ki-*ras*, c-Ha-*ras*, and c-*myc* in specific cell types during hepatocarcinogenesis. *Mol. Cell. Biol.,* 5:780–786.

Advances in Viral Oncology, Volume 6, edited by
George Klein, Raven Press, New York © 1987.

Development and Suppression of Malignancy

Leo Sachs

Department of Genetics, Weizmann Institute of Science, Rehovot 76100, Israel

In normal cells, multiplication and differentiation are controlled by different regulatory molecules. These regulators have to interact to achieve the correct balance between cell multiplication and differentiation during embryogenesis and during the subsequent normal functioning of the individual. The origin and further progression of malignancy result from genetic changes that uncouple the normal balance between multiplication and differentiation, resulting in the presence of too many growing cells. This uncoupling can occur in various ways (52,53,55,56). What are the changes that occur to uncouple normal controls and thereby produce cells with differing degrees of malignancy? When cells have become malignant, can malignancy then be suppressed, thus reverting malignant cells to nonmalignant cells? In malignant cells, abnormalities in the controls for multiplication and differentiation can vary. Do all abnormalities have to be corrected? Can they be bypassed in order to suppress malignancy? To answer these questions, I shall discuss results obtained from studies with normal and leukemic myeloid hematopoietic cells and some solid tumors as model systems.

NORMAL GROWTH FACTORS AND DIFFERENTIATION FACTORS

An understanding of the mechanisms that control multiplication (growth) and differentiation in normal cells is essential to elucidate the origin and reversibility of malignancy. The development of appropriate cell culture systems has made it possible to identify the normal regulators of growth (growth factors) for various types of cells and in some cell types, the normal regulators of differentiation (differentiation factors). This approach has been particularly fruitful in identifying the normal growth factors for all the different types of hematopoietic cells; first for myeloid cells (10,21,25,44,45) then for other cell types, including T lymphocytes (39) and B lymphocytes (40). The growth and differentiation factors of hematopoietic cells are different proteins that can be secreted by the cells that produce them. The normal differentiation factors, but not the growth factors, for myeloid cells are DNA-binding proteins (69). It will be interesting to determine how far this applies to normal differentiation factors for other cell types.

In cells of the myeloid series, four different growth-inducing proteins have been identified. These are now called macrophage and granulocyte inducers: type 1

(MGI-1), or colony-stimulating factors (CSF) (38,52,53,57). Of the four growth factors, one protein (M) induces the development of clones with both macrophages, another (G) clones with granulocytes, the third (GM) clones with both macrophages and granulocytes, and the fourth (also called interleukin-3, IL-3) clones with macrophages, granulocytes, eosinophils, mast cells, erythroid cells, and megakaryocytes (Table 1). Cloning the genes for the IL-3 (20,71) and GM (23) growth factors has shown that these two genes are completely unrelated in their nucleotide sequence. This multigene family represents a hierarchy of growth factors for various stages of hematopoietic cell development as the precursor cells become more restricted in their developmental program. It can be assumed that in the normal developmental program, IL-3 functions as a growth factor at an early stage when the precursors have the potential to develop into six cell types, GM at a later stage when the precursors have a more limited potential and can develop into two cell types, and G and M are growth factors when the developmental potential is still more restricted producing only one cell type. There is presumably a similar hierarchy of growth factors in the developmental program of other types of cells as well.

How do normal myeloid precursor cells, induced to multiply by these growth factors, develop into clones that contain mature differentiated cells that stop multiplying when they terminally differentiate? It appears unlikely that a growth factor that induces cell multiplication is also a differentiation factor whose action includes the stopping of cell multiplication in mature cells. Proteins that act as myeloid cell differentiation factors have been identified, and these have been called MGI-2, or differentiation factors (DF) (43,52,53,57,65). Experiments with normal myeloid cell precursors have shown that in these cells, the growth factors induce growth (cell viability and multiplication) and the production of differentiation factors (33,34,52,53) (Fig. 1). Myeloid differentiation factors induce differentiation directly, whereas growth factors induce differentiation indirectly by inducing the production of differentiation factors (Table 1). This induction of differentiation

TABLE 1. *Growth and differentiation factors in the development of myeloid hematopoietic cells*

Factor	Nomenclature	Differentiated Cell type affected	Induction of differentiation	
			Direct	Indirect[a]
Growth	MGI-M = M-CSF = CSF-1	Macrophages	−	+
	MGI-1G = G-CSF	Granulocytes	−	+
	MGI-1GM = GM-CSF	Macrophages and granulocytes	−	+
			−	+
	IL-3	Macrophages, granulocytes, and others		
Differentiation	MGI-2 = DF	Macrophages and granulocytes	+	−
			+	−

[a]Growth factor induces production of differentiation factor.

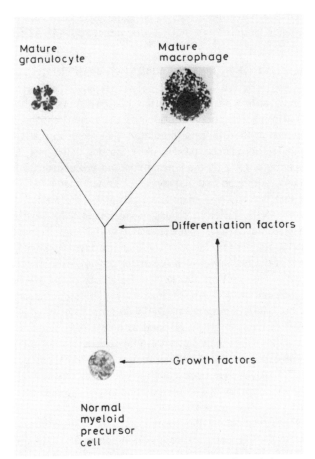

FIG. 1. Growth of normal myeloid precursor cells and their differentiation to macrophages or granulocytes are induced by different proteins; those that are growth factors and others that are differentiation factors. Growth factors induce cell viability and multiplication of the normal precursors and production in these cells of differentiation factors. This induction of differentiation factor by growth factor provides a coupling mechanism between the multiplication of normal precursors and their differentiation.

factors by growth factors thus ensures the normal coupling of growth and differentiation, a coupling mechanism that may also apply to other cell types. Differences in the time of the "switch-on" of differentiation factors would produce variations in the amount of cell multiplication before differentiation: There is more than one type of differentiation factor (55). Different growth factors may switch on different differentiation factors, which may determine the differentiated cell type. The results thus show that there are different proteins that participate in the developmental program of myeloid cells, growth factors and differentiation factors, and that growth factors can induce the synthesis of differentiation factors in normal myeloid precursors. In addition to their production by normal myeloid precursors, differentiation factors can also be produced by some other cell types and can induce differentiation when supplied externally to the target cells (43,52,53,55,57).

UNCOUPLING OF NORMAL CONTROLS

Identification of normal growth and differentiation factors and the cells that produce them has also made it possible to identify the various changes in the production of or response to these normal regulators that occur in malignancy. Normal myeloid growth factors can be produced by various cell types; however, these growth factors are not made by the normal myeloid precursors (33,34), so that the normal precursors require an external source of growth factor for cell viability and growth. Cells that become malignant have escaped some normal control, and in myeloid leukemic cells, different clones of malignant cells have been identified that show the possible changes that can occur in the normal response to growth and differentiation factors (51–53,55). There are different leukemic clones that (a) are independent of the normal growth factor for growth; (b) constitutively produce their own growth factor; (c) are blocked in the ability of growth factor to induce production of differentiation factor; (d) are changed in their requirement for normal growth factor but can still respond normally to normal differentiation factor; and (e) are defective in their ability to respond to normal differentiation factor. Cells blocked in the ability of growth factor to induce production of differentiation factor include some cell lines in culture that require an external source of growth factor for growth (33,34), and in some leukemic cells that constitutively produce their own growth factor, changes in specific components of the culture medium can restore the ability of growth factor to induce differentiation factor (57,63). There are thus various ways to uncouple the normal controls of growth and differentiation and various ways for the cells to become malignant. The uncoupling of normal controls and the various ways for cells to become malignant have been associated with changes from an induced to a constitutive expression of certain genes (11,29,52). The various types of changes that have been found in myeloid leukemic cells can serve as a model system to identify the different changes that give rise to malignant cells.

Growth factors induce cell viability and cell multiplication (33,34,66). Independence from normal growth factor or constitutive production of their own growth factor can also explain the survival and growth of metastasizing malignant cells in places in the body where growth factor required for survival of normal cells is not present. In cells that are malignant and that may still need some growth factor, the organ preference of metastasis could be due to production of the required growth factor in the organ where the metastasis occurs. Changes in response to chemotactic stimuli may also play a role in metastasis. Normal macrophages, granulocytes, and other cell types move in certain directions in response to various chemotactic stimuli; however, the myeloid leukemic cells that metastasize did not respond to these chemotactic stimuli (62). A decrease or lack of response to chemotactic stimuli that are presumably produced in certain organs could also explain the ability of metastatic and nonmetastatic tumor cells to move in a more disorganized manner than normal cells.

The transformation of normal cells to malignant cells requires a number of genetic changes, and the genes involved in the expression of malignancy are now called oncogenes (5,12,28). The change of normal genes to oncogenes are in all cases associated with changes in the structure or regulation of the normal genes. As is the case with normal genes, not all oncogenes have the same function. The *sis* oncogene is derived from a normal gene for platelet-derived growth factor (15,67), the *erb* B oncogene from the gene for the receptor for epidermal growth factor (16), the *erb* A oncogene from the gene for carbonic anhydrase that is involved in erythroid differentiation (14); and the *fms* proto-oncogene is related to the receptor for one of the hematopoietic growth factors (58) (CSF-1 = MGI-1M = M-CSF; Table 1). These studies are thus providing further information on the genetic differences that result in changes in the normal production and response to growth and differentiation factors that occur in malignancy. The origin and progression of malignancy can involve different genetic changes, including changes in gene dosage (50), gene mutations, deletions, and gene rearrangements (27,28). Various genetic changes in the structure or regulation of the normal genes that control growth and differentiation can thus produce, in different ways, the uncoupling of the normal controls which is required for the origin and further progression of malignancy.

INDUCTION OF DIFFERENTIATION IN MALIGNANT CELLS

The various types of myeloid leukemic cells include clones that have changed their normal requirement for growth factor and in which growth factor no longer switches on the production of differentiation factor but which can still be induced to differentiate to mature nondividing cells by normal differentiation factors. These clones, which are called D^+ clones for differentiation, can be induced to differentiate normally to mature macrophages and granulocytes, via the normal sequence of gene expression that occurs during differentiation, by incubation of the cells with normal differentiation factor (50,53). The mature cells, which can be formed from all the cells of a leukemic clone, then stop multiplying like normal mature cells and are no longer malignant. Experiments carried out in animals have shown that normal differentiation of these myeloid leukemic cells to mature nondividing cells can be induced not only *in vitro* but *in vivo* as well (22,31,32,35,36,68). These leukemias therefore grow progressively when there are too many leukemic cells for the normal amount of differentiation factor in the body. The development of leukemia can be inhibited in mice with these leukemic cells by increasing the normal amount of differentiation factor by either injecting it or injecting a compound that increases production of differentiation factor by cells in the body (32,35).

The culture of different clones of myeloid leukemic cells in the presence of differentiation factor has shown that in addition to D^+ clones, there are also differentiation-defective D^- clones. Some of those clones were induced to an intermediate stage of differentiation, which then slows down the growth of the cells; others could not be induced to differentiate, even to this intermediate stage (30,50,51,53) (Fig. 2). Since normal differentiation factor can induce differentiation to mature nondividing cells in the D^+ clones, it can be suggested that D^+ clones are the early stages of leukemia and that the formation of the different types of D^- clones may represent later stages in the further progression of malignancy. Does this progression include complete loss of the genes for differentiation in D^- clones? To answer this, experiments were carried out to determine whether compounds other than normal differentiation factor can induce differentiation in myeloid leukemic cells.

Studies with a variety of chemicals other than normal differentiation-inducing protein have shown that many compounds can induce differentiation in D^+ clones of myeloid leukemic cells. These include certain steroid hormones, chemicals, such as cytosine arabinoside, adriamycin, methotrexate, and other chemicals that are used today in cancer chemotherapy; and x-ray irradiation. At high doses, these compounds, used in cancer therapy, and x-ray irradiation kill cells, whereas at low doses they can induce differentiation. Not all these compounds are equally active on the same leukemic clone. A variety of chemicals can also induce differentiation in clones that are not induced to differentiate by normal differentiation factor; in some clones, induction of differentiation requires combined treatment with differ-

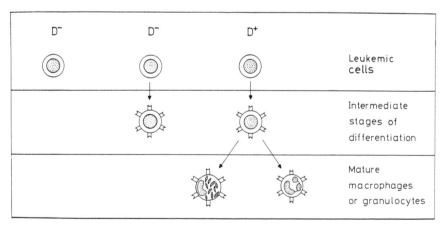

FIG. 2. Classification of different types of clones of myeloid leukemic cells according to their ability to be induced to differentiate by normal differentiation factor. Some differentiation-defective (D^-) clones can be induced by normal differentiation factor to intermediate stages of differentiation, whereas other D^- clones were not induced to differentate by this factor, even to an intermediate stage.

ent compounds (51,53,55). The results show that although the response for induction of differentiation by differentiation factor has been altered, the D^- clones have not lost all the genes for differentiation. In addition to certain steroids and chemicals used today in chemotherapy and irradiation, other compounds that can induce differentiation in myeloid leukemic cells include insulin, bacterial lipopolysaccharide, certain plant lectins, and phorbol esters, with or without differentiation factor (51,55). It is probable that all myeloid leukemic cells no longer susceptible to normal differentiation factor alone can be induced to differentiate by the appropriate combination of compounds.

The ability of a variety of compounds to induce differentiation in malignant cells is not restricted to myeloid leukemic cells. Erythroleukemic cells can be induced to differentiate by various chemicals (19,37). Erythroprotein, a normal protein that induces the production of hemoglobin in normal erythrocytes, did not induce hemoglobin in these erythroleukemias. These erythroleukemias are thus like D^- myeloid leukemias that are not induced to differentiate by the normal myeloid differentiation factor. It has also been shown that some of the compounds that induce differentiation in leukemic cells can induce differentiation in tumors derived from other types of cells (37).

DIFFERENT PATHWAYS FOR INDUCING DIFFERENTIATION

Studies on the way in which different compounds act in myeloid leukemic cells have shown that there are different pathways for inducing differentiation. Some compounds induce differentiation by inducing the production of differentiation-inducing protein in the D^+ leukemic cells, whereas others, such as the steroid hormones, induce differentiation without inducing this protein. Various compounds can also induce differentiation in D^- clones that are not induced to differentiate by normal differentiation factor. Not all clones respond to the same compound, and in some clones differentiation requires combined treatment with more than one compound. Not all compounds act in the same way, and in cases of combined treatment, each compound induces changes not induced by the other. The combined treatment then produces, by complementation, the appropriate gene expression that is required for differentiation (53,55).

Further evidence that there are different pathways of inducing differentiation in leukemic cells was obtained from studies on changes in the synthesis of cellular proteins in normal myeloid precursors and different types of myeloid leukemic cells (11,29,52). These experiments have shown that there are protein changes that have to be induced in normal cells and are constitutive in leukemic cells. The leukemic cells were found to be constitutive for changes in the synthesis of a group of proteins that were only induced in the normal cells after the addition of growth factor. These protein changes, which include the appearance of some proteins and disappearance of others, were constitutive in all the leukemic clones studied derived from different leukemias. They have been called constitutive in leukemia

(C_{leuk}); D^+ leukemic cells can be induced to differentiate to mature cells by normal differentiation factor. This showed that the differentiation program induced by differentiation factor can proceed normally, even when the protein changes induced in normal cells by growth factor have become constitutive. There were other protein changes that were induced by differentiation factor in normal and D^+ leukemic clones but were constitutive in the differentiation-defective D^- leukemic clones. With this group of proteins, the most differentiation-defective clones showed the highest number of constitutive protein changes. These protein changes have been called (C_{def}), constitutive in differentiation defective (29,52) (Fig. 3).

The protein changes during differentiation of normal myeloid precursors are induced as a series of parallel multiple pathways of gene expression. It can be assumed that normal differentiation requires synchronous initiation and progression of these multiple parallel pathways. The presence of constitutive instead of induced gene expression for some pathways can be expected to produce asynchrony in the coordination required for differentiation. Depending on the pathways involved, this asynchrony can then produce blocks in the induction and termination of the differentiation program (11,29,52). D^- leukemic cells can be treated so as to induce the reversion of C_{def} proteins from the constitutive to the induced state. This reversion was associated with restoration of inducibility for differentiation by the normal differentiation factor. Reversion from the constitutive to the induced state in these cells thus restored the synchrony of gene expression that is required for differentiation (64).

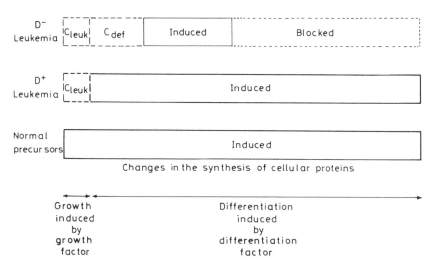

FIG. 3. Schematic summary of changes in the synthesis of cellular proteins associated with growth and differentiation: (C_{leuk}), constitutive expression of changes in all the clones of myeloid leukemic cells compared to normal myeloblasts; (C_{def}), constitutive expression of changes in differentiation-defective (D^-) clones of leukemic cells compared to differentiation-competent (D^+) leukemic clones and normal myeloblasts. The most differentiation-defective D^- clones (Fig. 2) showed the highest number of C_{def} constitutive protein changes (29).

The study of different mutants of myeloid leukemic cells has shown that in addition to the existence of constitutive protein changes that inhibit differentiation of myeloid leukemic cells by normal differentiation factor, there are also constitutive protein changes that inhibit differentiation by the steroid hormone dexamethasone. The constitutive changes that inhibit differentiation by dexamethasone are different from those that inhibit differentiation by normal differentiation factor (11). These experiments have thus identified different pathways of gene expression for inducing differentiation and have also shown that genetic changes that block differentiation by one compound need not affect differentiation by another compound that uses alternative pathways. Since the normal differentiation factor for myeloid cells has been identified and leukemic clones have been found that respond to this normal differentiation factor, it was possible to compare the ability of clones of myeloid leukemic cells to be induced to differentiate by the normal inducer and by other compounds. Even though the normal differentiation factors for many other cell types have not yet been identified, it seems likely that the conclusions on the different pathways of inducing differentiation derived from studies with myeloid leukemic cells will also apply to other types of tumors.

ONCOGENE SUPPRESSORS AND BYPASSING OF GENETIC DEFECTS IN THE SUPPRESSION OF MALIGNANCY

The change of cells from normal to malignant involves a sequence of genetic changes. Evidence has, however, been obtained with various types of tumors, including sarcomas (50), myeloid leukemias (50,51), and teratocarcinomas (61), that malignant cells have not lost the genes that control normal growth and differentiation. This was first shown in sarcomas by the finding that it was possible to reverse the phenotype from malignant to nonmalignant with a high frequency in cloned sarcoma cells whose malignancy had been induced by chemical carcinogens, by x-ray irradiation, or by a tumor-inducing virus (46,47,50). In sarcomas induced after transformation of normal fibroblasts in culture with chemical carcinogens (3,4) or x-ray irradiation (8,9), this reversibility of malignancy included reversion to the limited life span found with normal fibroblasts (48).

Chromosome studies on normal fibroblasts, sarcomas, revertants from sarcomas that had regained a nonmalignant phenotype, and re-revertants showed that the difference between these malignant and nonmalignant cells is controlled by the balance between genes for expression (E) and genes for suppression (S) of malignancy (6,7,24,47,50,70). When there is enough suppression to neutralize expression, malignancy is suppressed; when the amount of suppression is not sufficient to neutralize expression, malignancy is expressed. These early experiments have shown (6,7,24,47,50,54,70) that in addition to genes for expression of malignancy (oncogenes or E genes), there are other genes (S genes), that are now called soncogenes (54), or antioncogenes (13) that can suppress the action of oncogenes. Suppression of the action of the Ki-*ras* oncogene in revertants (13,42) is presumably due to such suppressor genes. The balance between oncogenes and their suppressors also seems to determine malignancy in other tumors, including human retinoblastomas (41).

In the mechanism found with sarcomas (50,54), reversion was obtained by chromosome segregation, resulting in a change in gene dosage due to a change in the balance of specific chromosomes. This suppression of malignancy by chromosome segregation, with a return to the gene balance required for expression of the nonmalignant phenotype, occurred without hybridization between different types of cells. The nonmalignant cells were thus derived from the malignant ones by genetic segregation. Suppression of malignancy associated with chromosome changes, including changes in gene balance, have also been found after hybridization between different types of cells (2,17,26,27,49,60). These studies on cell hybrids have led to similar conclusions to those obtained from the reversal of malignancy in sarcomas without hybridization between different cell types.

In addition to this reversion of malignancy by chromosome segregation, another mechanism of reversion was found in myeloid leukemia. These leukemic cells also have an abnormal chromosome composition (1). In this second mechanism, a high frequency of reversion to a nonmalignant phenotype was also obtained in certain clones, but unlike the mechanism found with sarcomas, this reversion was not associated with chromosome segregation. Phenotypic reversion of malignancy in these leukemic cells was obtained by induction of the normal sequence of cell differentiation by normal differentiation factor (50–53). In this reversion of the malignant phenotype, stopping cell multiplication by inducing differentiation to mature cells bypasses genetic changes in the requirement for normal growth factor and the block in the ability of growth factor to induce differentiation factor that produced the malignant phenotype. Genetic changes that make cells defective in their ability to be induced to differentiate by the normal differentiation factor occur in the evolution of myeloid leukemia; but even these cells can be induced to differentiate by other compounds, either singly or in combination, that can induce the differentiation program by other pathways (50,52,55). Also in these cases, stopping cell multiplication by inducing differentiation by these alternative pathways bypasses the genetic changes that block response to the normal differentiation factor. This bypassing of genetic defects is also presumably the mechanism by which malignancy is suppressed by inducing differentiation in other types of tumors, such as erythroleukemias and neuroblastomas. It is also possible that all oncogenes are lost (18) or that the change of normal genes to oncogenes is actually reversed.

Studies on the chromosomes of myeloid leukemic cells have shown that the change from D^- to D^+ and *vice versa,* i.e., the ability to be induced to differentiate to mature nondividing cells by normal differentiation factor, is controlled by the balance between genes that allow induction of differentiation and genes that suppress differentiation (1). It has also been shown in cell hybrids, that chromosome changes resulting in changes in gene balance can suppress malignancy by restoring the ability of the cells to be induced to differentiate to non-dividing cells *in vivo* in a location in the body where the cells are exposed to what is presumably

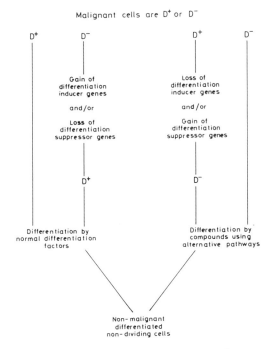

Malignant cells are D⁺ or D⁻

FIG. 4. Suppression of malignancy by inducing differentiation can be achieved in different ways. Malignant cells can (D⁺) or can not (D⁻) be induced to differentiate by normal differentiation factors to mature nondividing cells. The D⁻ cells can, however, be induced to differentiate by other compounds that induce differentiation by alternative pathways. Chromosome changes, that change the balance between genes for induction and genes for suppression of differentiation, can change cells from D⁻ to D⁺ and *vice versa.*

the normal differentiation factor (59). The appropriate chromosome changes thus also change these hybrid cells from D⁻ to D⁺. The same may possibly apply to the revertants of sarcoma cells that multiply in culture and are nonmalignant *in vivo* which have been obtained without hybridization. Chromosome changes can thus change malignant cells from D⁻ to D⁺, so that the cells can then be induced to differentiate when exposed to normal differentiation factors (Fig. 4).

It can therefore be concluded that expression of malignancy due to changes of normal genes to oncogenes is not irreversible; malignancy can again be suppressed. Results on the reversibility of malignancy have shown that (a) there are various ways of suppressing malignancy; (b) reversion does not have to restore all of the normal controls; and (c) the stopping of cell multiplication by inducing differentiation can bypass genetic abnormalities that give rise to malignancy.

SUMMARY

The identification of normal growth and differentiation factors and how they interact in normal development has made it possible to identify the mechanisms that uncouple growth and differentiation in the development and progression of malignancy. When cells have become malignant, the malignant phenotype can again be suppressed. Results on the reversibility of malignancy have shown that in addition to genes for the expression of malignancy (oncogenes), there are other genes (called soncogenes or antioncogenes) that can suppress the action of oncogenes, that reversion does not have to restore all the normal controls, and that stopping cell multiplication by inducing differentiation to mature cells can bypass the genetic abnormalities that give rise to malignancy. Tumor formation can thus be suppressed by either correcting or bypassing the genetic abnormalities that produce malignant cells.

ACKNOWLEDGMENTS

This research is now supported by the National Foundation for Cancer Research, Bethesda; the Jerome A. and Estelle R. Newman Assistance Fund; Julian Wallerstein Foundation; and the Farleigh S. Dickinson Jr. Foundation.

REFERENCES

1. Azumi, J., and Sachs, L. (1977): Chromosome mapping of the genes that control differentiation and malignancy in myeloid leukemic cells. *Proc. Natl. Acad. Sci. U.S.A.*, 74:253–257.
2. Benedict, W.F., Weissman, B.E., Mark, C., and Stanbridge, E.J. (1984): Tumorigenicity of human HT1080 fibrosarcoma × normal fibroblast hybrids: Chromosome dosage dependency. *Cancer Res.*, 44:3471–3479.
3. Berwald, Y., and Sachs, L. (1963): *In vitro* cell transformation with chemical carcinogens. *Nature*, 200:1182–1184.
4. Berwald, Y., and Sachs, L. (1965): *In vitro* transformation of normal cells to tumor cells by carcinogenic hydrocarbons. *J. Natl. Cancer Inst.*, 35:641–661.
5. Bishop, J.M. (1983): Cellular oncogenes and retroviruses. *Ann. Rev. Biochem.*, 52:301–354.
6. Bloch-Shtacher, N., and Sachs, L. (1976): Chromosome balance and the control of malignancy. *J. Cell. Physiol.*, 87:89–100.
7. Bloch-Shtacher, N., and Sachs, L. (1977): Identification of a chromosome that controls malignancy in Chinese hamster cells. *J. Cell. Physiol.*, 93:205–212.
8. Borek, C., and Sachs, L. (1966): *In vitro* cell transformation by x-irradiation. *Nature*, 210:276–278.
9. Borek, C., and Sachs, L. (1967): Cell susceptibility to transformation by x-irradiation and fixation of the transformed state. *Proc. Natl. Acad. Sci. U.S.A.*, 57:1522–1527.
10. Bradley, T.R., and Metcalf, D. (1966): The growth of mouse bone marrow cells *in vitro*. *Aust. J. Exp. Biol. Med. Sci.*, 44:287–300.
11. Cohen, L., and Sachs, L. (1981): Constitutive gene expression in myeloid leukemia and cell competence for induction of differentiation by the steroid dexamethasone. *Proc. Natl. Acad. Sci. U.S.A.*, 78:353–357.
12. Cooper, G.M. (1982): Cellular transforming genes. *Science*, 218:801–806.
13. Craig, R.W., and Sager, R. (1985): Suppression of tumorigenicity in hybrids of normal and oncogene-transformed CHEF cells. *Proc. Natl. Acad. Sci. U.S.A.*, 82:2062–2066.
14. Debuire, B., Henry, C., Benaissa, M., Biserte, G., Claverie, J.M., Saule, S., Martin, P., and Stehelin, D. (1984): Sequencing the *erb* A gene of avian erythroblastosis virus reveals a new type of oncogene. *Science*, 224:1456–1459.
15. Doolittle, R.F., Hunkapiller, M.W., Hood, L.E., Devare, S.G., Robbins, K.C., Aaronson, S.A., and Antoniades, H.N. (1983): Simian sarcoma virus oncogene, v-*sis*, is derived from the gene (or genes) encoding a platelet-derived growth factor. *Science*, 221:275–277.
16. Downward, J., Yarden, Y., Mayers, E., Scrace, G., Totty, N., Stockwell, P., Ulrich, A., Schlessinger, J., and Waterfield, M.D. (1984): Close similarity of epidermal growth factor receptor and v-*erb*-B oncogene protein sequences. *Nature*, 307:521–527.
17. Evans, E.P., Burtenshaw, M.D., Brown, B.B., Hennion, R., and Harris, H. (1982): The analysis of malignancy by cell fusion. X. Reexamination and clarification of the cytogenetic problem. *J. Cell Sci.*, 56:113–130.
18. Frankel, A.E., Haapala, D.K., Newbouer, R.L., and Fischinger, P.J. (1976): Elimination of the sarcoma genome from murine sarcoma virus-transformed cat cells. *Science*, 191:1264–1266.
19. Friend, C. (1978): The phenomenon of differentiation in murine erythroleukemic cells. *Harvey Lect.*, 72:253–281.
20. Fung, M.C., Hapel, S.J., Ymer, S., Cohen, D.R., Johnson, R.M., Campbell, H.D., and Young, I.G. (1984): Molecular cloning of cDNA for murine interleukin-3. *Nature*, 307:233–237.

21. Ginsburg, H., and Sachs, L. (1963): Formation of pure suspension of mast cells in tissue culture by differentiation of lymphoid cells from the mouse thymus. *J. Natl. Cancer Inst.*, 31:1–40.
22. Gootwine, E., Webb, C.G., and Sachs, L. (1982): Participation of myeloid leukemic cells injected into embryos in hematopoietic differentiation in adult mice. *Nature*, 299:63–65.
23. Gough, N.M., Gough, J., Metcalf, D., Kelson, A., Grail, D., Nicola, N.A., Burgess, A.W., and Dunn, A.R. (1984): Molecular cloning of cDNA encoding a murine haematopoietic growth regulator, granulocyte-macrophage colony-stimulating factor. *Nature*, 309:763–767.
24. Hitotsumachi, S., Rabinowitz, Z., and Sachs, L. (1971): Chromosomal control of reversion in transformed cells. *Nature*, 231:511–514.
25. Ichikawa, Y., Pluznik, D.H., and Sachs, L. (1966): *In vitro* control of the development of macrophage and granulocyte colonies. *Proc. Natl. Acad. Sci. U.S.A.*, 56:488–495.
26. Kitchin, R.M., Gadi, I.K., Smith, B.L., and Sager, R. (1982): Genetic analysis of tumorogenesis. X. Chromosome studies of transformed mutants and tumor-derived CHEF/18 cells. *Somat. Cell Genet.*, 8:677–689.
27. Klein, G. (1981): The role of gene dosage and genetic transposition in carcinogenesis. *Nature*, 194:313–318.
28. Land, H., Parada, L.F., and Weinberg, R.A. (1983): Cellular oncogenes and multistep carcinogenesis. *Science*, 222:771–778.
29. Liebermann, D., Hoffman-Liebermann, B., and Sachs, L. (1980): Molecular dissection of differentiation in normal and leukemic myeloblasts: Separately programmed pathways of gene expression. *Dev. Biol.*, 79:46–63.
30. Lotem, J., and Sachs, L. (1974): Different blocks in the differentiation of myeloid leukemic cells. *Proc. Natl. Acad. Sci. U.S.A.*, 71:3507–3511.
31. Lotem, J., and Sachs, L. (1978): *In vivo* induction of normal differentiation in myeloid leukemic cells. *Proc. Natl. Acad. Sci. U.S.A.*, 75:3781–3785.
32. Lotem, J., and Sachs, L. (1981): *In vivo* inhibition of the development of myeloid leukemia by injection of macrophage- and granulocyte-inducing protein. *Int. J. Cancer*, 28:375–386.
33. Lotem, J., and Sachs, L. (1982): Mechanisms that uncouple growth and differentiation in myeloid leukemia cells. Restoration of requirement for normal growth-inducing protein without restoring induction of differentiation-inducing protein. *Proc. Natl. Acad. Sci. U.SA.*, 79:4347–4351.
34. Lotem, J., and Sachs, L. (1983): Coupling of growth and differentiation in normal myeloid precursors and the breakdown of this coupling in leukemia. *Int. J. Cancer*, 32:127–134.
35. Lotem, J., and Sachs, L. (1984): Control of *in vivo* differentiation of myeloid leukemic cells. IV. Inhibition of leukemia development by myeloid differentiation-inducing protein. *Int. J. Cancer*, 33:147–154.
36. Lotem, J., and Sachs, L. (1986): Control of *in vivo* differentiation of myeloid leukemic cells. V. Regulation by response to antigen. *Leuk. Res.*, 9:1479–1486.
37. Marks, P., and Rifkind, R.A. (1978): Erythroleukemia differentiation. *Annu. Rev. Biochem.*, 47:419–448.
38. Metcalf, D. (1985): The granulocyte-macrophage colony-stimulating factors. *Science*, 299:16–22.
39. Mier, J.W., and Gallo, R.C. (1980): Purification and some characteristics of human T-cell growth factor from phytohemagglutinin-stimulated lymphocyte-conditioned media. *Proc. Natl. Acad. Sci. U.S.A.*, 77:6134–6138.
40. Möller, G. (ed.) (1984): B-cell growth and differentiation factors. *Immunol. Rev.*, 78.
41. Murphree, A.L., and Benedict, W.P. (1984): Retinoblastoma: Clues to human oncogenesis. *Science*, 223:1028–1033.
42. Noda, M., Selinger, Z., Scolnick, E.M., and Bassin, R.H. (1983): Flat revertants isolated from Kirsten sarcoma virus-transformed cells are resistant to the action of specific oncogenes. *Proc. Natl. Acad. Sci. U.S.A.*, 80:5602–5606.
43. Olsson, I., Sarngadharan, M.G., Breitman, T.R., and Gallo, R.C. (1984): Isolation and characterisation of a T-lymphocyte-derived differentiation-inducing factor for the myeloid leukemic cell line HL-60. *Blood*, 63:510–517.
44. Pluznik, D.H., and Sachs, L. (1965): The cloning of normal "mast" cells in tissue culture. *J. Cell. Comp. Physiol.*, 66:319–324.
45. Pluznik, D.H., and Sachs, L. (1966): The induction of clones of normal "mast" cells by a substance from conditioned medium. *Exp. Cell. Res.*, 43:553–563.
46. Rabinowitz, Z., and Sachs, L. (1968): Reversion of properties in cells transformed by polyoma virus. *Nature*, 220:1203–1206.
47. Rabinowitz, Z., and Sachs, L. (1970): Control of the reversion of properties in transformed cells. *Nature*, 225:136–139.

48. Rabinowitz, Z., and Sachs, L. (1970): The formation of variants with a reversion of properties of transformed cells. V. Reversion to a limited life span. *Int. J. Cancer*, 6:388–398.
49. Ringertz, N.R., and Savage, R.E. (1976): *Cell Hybrids*. Academic Press, New York.
50. Sachs, L. (1974): Regulation of membrane changes, differentiation and malignancy in carcinogenesis. *Harvey Lect.*, 68:1–35.
51. Sachs, L. (1978): Control of normal cell differentiation and the phenotypic reversion of malignancy in myeloid leukemia. *Nature*, 274:535–539.
52. Sachs, L. (1980): Constitutive uncoupling of pathways of gene expression that control growth and differentiation in myeloid leukemia: A model for the origin and progression of malignancy. *Proc. Natl. Acad. Sci. U.S.A.*, 77:6153–6156.
53. Sachs, L. (1982): Normal developmental programmes in myeloid leukaemia: Regulatory proteins in the control of growth and differentiation. *Cancer Surveys*, 1:321–342.
54. Sachs, L. (1984): Normal regulators, oncogenes, and the reversibility of malignancy. *Cancer Surveys*, 3:210–228.
55. Sachs, L. (1985): Regulators of growth, differentiation, and the reversion of malignancy. Normal hematopoiesis and leukemia. In: *Molecular Biology of Tumor Cells, Nobel Symposium*, edited by B. Wahren, G. Holm, S. Hammarströhm, and P. Perlmann, pp. 257–280, Raven Press, New York.
56. Sachs, L. (1986): Growth, differentiation and the reversal of malignancy. *Sci. Am.*, 254:40–47.
57. Sachs, L., and Lotem, J. (1984): Haematopoietic growth factors. *Nature*, 312:407.
58. Sherr, C.J., Rettenmier, C.W., Sacca, R., Roussel, M.F., Look, A.T., and Stanley, E.R. (1985): The c-*fms* proto-oncogene product is related to the receptor for the mononuclear phagocyte growth factor CSF-1. *Cell*, 41:665–676.
59. Stanbridge, E.J. (1984): Genetic analysis of tumorogenicity in human cell hybrids. *Cancer Surv.*, 3:334–350.
60. Stanbridge, E.J., Der, C.J., Doersen, C-J., Nishimi, R.Y., Peehl, D.M., Weissman, B.E., and Wilkinson, J.E. (1982): Human cell hybrids: Analysis of transformation and tumorigenicity. *Science*, 215:252–259.
61. Stewart, T.A., and Mintz, B. (1981): Successive generations of mice produced from an established culture line of euploid teratocarcinoma cells. *Proc. Natl. Acad. Sci. U.S.A.*, 78:6314–6318.
62. Symonds, G., and Sachs, L. (1979): Activation of normal genes in malignant cells: Activation of chemotaxis in relation to other stages of normal differentiation in myeloid leukemia. *Somatic Cell Genet.*, 5:931–944.
63. Symonds, G., and Sachs, L. (1982): Autoinduction of differentiation in myeloid leukemic cells: Restoration of normal coupling between growth and differentiation in leukemic cells that constitutively produce their own growth-inducing protein. *EMBO J.*, 1:1343–1346.
64. Symonds, G., and Sachs, L. (1983): Synchrony of gene expression and the differentiation of myeloid leukemic cells: Reversion from constitutive to inducible protein synthesis. *EMBO J.*, 2:663–667.
65. Tomida, M., Yamamoto-Kamaguchi, Y., and Hozumi, M. (1984): Purification of a factor inducing differentiation of mouse myeloid leukemic M1 cells from conditioned medium from mouse fibroblast L929 cells. *J. Biol. Chem.*, 259:10978–10982.
66. Tushinski, R.J., Oliver, I.T., Guilbert, L.J., Tynan, P.W., Warner, J.R., and Stanley, E.R. (1982): Survival of mononuclear phagocytes depends on a lineage-specific growth factor that the differentiated cells selectively destroy. *Cell*, 208:71–81.
67. Waterfield, M.D., Scrace, G.T., Whittle, N., Stroobant, P., Johnsson, A., Wasteson, A., Westermark, B., Heldin, C.H., Huang, J.S., and Deuel, T.F. (1983): Platelet-derived growth factor is structurally related to the putative transforming protein p28^{sis} of simian sarcoma virus. *Nature*, 304:35–39.
68. Webb, C.G., Gootwine, E., and Sachs, L. (1984): Developmental potential of myeloid leukemia cells injected into mid-gestation embryos. *Dev. Biol.*, 101:221–224.
69. Weisinger, G., and Sachs, L. (1983): DNA-binding protein that induces cell differentiation. *EMBO J.*, 2:2105–2107.
70. Yamamoto, T., Rabinowitz, Z., and Sachs, L. (1973): Identification of the chromosomes that control malignancy. *Nature New Biol.*, 243:247–250.
71. Yokota, T., Lee, F., Rennick, D., Hall, C., Arai, N., Mosmann, T., Nabel, G., Cantor, H., and Arai, K.-I. (1984): Isolation and characterization of a mouse cDNA clone that expresses mast-cell growth-factor activity in monkey cells. *Proc. Natl. Acad. Sci. U.S.A.*, 81:1070–1074.

Advances in Viral Oncology, Volume 6, edited by
George Klein, Raven Press, New York © 1987.

Oncogenes, Genetic Instability, and Evolution of the Metastatic Phenotype

Garth L. Nicolson

Department of Tumor Biology, The University of Texas M.D. Anderson Hospital and Tumor Institute, Houston, Texas 77030

The progression of cancer to the metastatic phenotype is probably the result of several sequential cellular changes that lead eventually to the selection and evolution of tumor cells with multiple genetic and possibly epigenetic modifications (17,69,94,95,100,101). Although Foulds (43) did not attempt to define tumor evolution or progression in genetic terms, he did note that these changes occurred irreversibly and independently and that they seemed to be unique to each tumor. Thus, the independent assortment of tumor properties is believed to create tumor variation. The idea that the malignant spread of tumors requires multiple changes in cellular properties and tumor variation is not unlike Fould's concepts.

The invasion and metastasis of tumor cells is known to occur via a complex series of sequential steps that require unique tumor cell characteristics and appropriate host properties (41,92,93,96–98,112,127). Paget (105) first proposed this concept as the "seed and soil" hypothesis, which states that the microenvironment of individual organs or tissues ("soil") must be appropriate for the implantation, survival, and growth of unique tumor cells ("seeds"). The nonrandom metastatic distributions and other properties of many clinical cancers support Paget's hypothesis and do not support the concept (151) that cancer dissemination is a strictly random process. If particular tumor cells with specific cellular properties are important in the metastatic process, then these characteristics should arise from unique genetic and epigenetic differences in malignant compared to benign tumor cells. This review shall focus on the possible role of these reported changes in generating the metastatic phenotype. Particular attention shall be paid to the possibility that modifications in oncogenes or proto-oncogenes or their expression could be the changes that lead eventually to or are characteristic of the generation of the metastatic phenotype.

TUMOR CELL HETEROGENEITY

One of the most interesting and potentially important features of highly malignant neoplasms is that they are composed of diverse cell populations that are heterogeneous in a variety of properties, including cell morphology, cell surface antigens, glycolipids and glycoproteins, cell adhesion and recognition components, synthetic and hydrolytic enzymes, cellular locomotion and response to tactic signals, and invasiveness and metastatic properties. Cellular heterogeneity is also a factor in therapeutic sensitivities to drugs, radiation, hyperthermia, and in host response mechanisms (40,54,57,59,92,93,96–98); however, cellular phenotypic heterogeneity is not strictly a property of malignant cells. Cellular population diversity occurs in normal cells and tissues, but in general, it is more pronounced in malignant than in benign or normal cells (109,110).

It is thought that even heterogeneous populations of malignant cells develop originally from a single cell (38,100). Evidence of cell clonal origin exists even in tumors that have undergone diversification to form heterogeneous cell populations (18,39,100,155). In the case of advanced malignancies, heterogeneity is thought to have been caused by the evolution or progression of malignant cell subpopulations within tumors. Foulds (43) studied this phenomenon in a series of spontaneous mammary tumors, and he found that they gradually and independently gained autonomy from host controls, such as hormone regulation. It is now thought that virtually any characteristic of neoplastic cells may be subject to independent variation, selection, and evolution, which lead eventually to tumors that are increasingly unlinked to host control and regulatory mechanisms (93,94,100,101). Nowell (100) proposed that gene alterations—genetic instability—can change the evolution or progression of tumors. As tumor cells acquire genetic changes, variants arise in the population, and as these variants proliferate, their progeny can evolve with properties that are the most favorable for their survival and growth despite various host and externally applied (therapeutic) pressures.

In addition to being different for each neoplasm, the rates of tumor evolution or progression may also vary during the natural history of the disease. In this scheme a benign tumor would have less tendency than a malignant tumor to progress and change phenotypically. Cell populations in the latter would be expected to diversify phenotypically at varying rates, some quickly generating highly metastatic and resistant tumor cell subpopulations (94,95,114).

The competitive tumor cell microenvironment may be important in phenotypic diversification of tumors and in the selection of variant tumor cells for enhanced survival and growth characteristics. For example, tumor cell subpopulations that are inhibited by host defenses or that are less capable of responding to microenvironmental signals, such as growth or differentiation factors, may change in importance within a tumor. Neoplastic cells that have competitive advantages over neighboring cells would eventually become the dominant population in such a scheme and evolve with particular cellular characteristics. Thus, it is likely that during the progression or evolution of tumors, variation occurs in the composition of tumor cell subpopulations. Even though such tumors may remain heterogeneous, their overall cellular characteristics may shift to those more favorable for their survival, growth, and malignancy. This is not to say that the progression of tumors leads necessarily to rapidly growing, highly malignant cells. Since these processes probably are governed to some degree by random events (such as random somatic mutations) and other changes, regression should also be possible, and in fact, tumor regression has been documented in certain rare cases. At the cellular level, the high reversion rates of many metastatic cell systems have led to proposals that a heterogeneous malignant cell population is maintaining a dynamic equilibrium (80).

Some changes in malignant tumor cells may be unrelated to progression and malignancy. Cellular properties that are unimportant to the malignant phenotype may, for example, be enhanced, diminished, or even lost at later stages of tumor progression. In some cases, the loss or reduction of tumor cell activities or components during progression has been interpreted as "loss of differentiation." The relationship of cellular differentiation to states of tumor progression and malignancy is unclear, however, and these characteristics may be only casually related (93,94).

ONCOGENES AND NEOPLASTIC TRANSFORMATION

The transforming genes of retroviruses (viral oncogenes or v-*onc*) and their cellular progenitors (proto-oncogenes, cellular oncogenes, or c-*onc*) are thought to be important elements in the neoplastic transformation of certain susceptible cells (24,146,149). Oncogenes and proto-oncogenes are highly conserved gene families (30) whose expression seems to be related to cellular growth and differentiation properties (12,76,88). They encode proteins that function abnormally and allow a cell to circumvent the normal controls that regulate cell growth (62,66), and possibly differentiation and other characteristics.

The aberrant structure or expression of proto-oncogenes or their abbreviated viral oncogene counterparts in neoplastic cells appears to be important in the transformation events of at least certain tumors. In virally transformed cells, the role of v-*onc* elements in neoplastic transformation is probably the least unambiguous role for these genes. For example, retroviruses can deliver to a susceptible target cell strong transforming v-*onc* genes, which when suitably incorporated in the host cell genome will cause neoplastic transformation in essentially one step. This type of rapid, dominant transformation event probably is not very relevant for human cancer, since viruses and their v-*onc* genes have been placed under severe selective pressures that are not likely to be encountered under natural conditions (140), and available evidence indicates that spontaneous human cancers probably arise by a stepwise rather than a "one-hit" process (17,69,70).

It is clear that human cancer does not usually result from activation of a single, dominantly acting oncogene. Fusion of malignant human cells with nonmalignant human cells results in suppression of tumorigenicity but not transformation properties in tissue culture (33). These results have led to speculation that antioncogenes (71) or tumor-suppressor (133) genes may control important events in the tumorigenic process. Support for this concept is that nontumorigenic hybrids of human HT1080 fibrosarcoma and normal human fibroblasts eventually evolve tumorigenic segregants that have lost specific chromosomes (chromosome 1 and possibly chromosome 4); however, they continue to synthesize *ras*-encoded p21, regardless of tumorigenic potential (8).

In some spontaneous cancers, the expression or activities of cellular oncogenes can be altered by a few general mechanisms that will eventually result in neoplastic transformation (10,46). For example, the expression of c-*onc* genes can be increased by gene amplification or chromosomal rearrangements, and these events can alter the growth characteristics of some normal cells. In addition, mutations in the coding regions of a proto-oncogene can cause functional alterations of the protein product without increased gene expression, resulting in aberrant cellular growth characteristics. It should be noted that many c-*onc* genes are, however, expressed regularly in normal cells without evidence of transforming capacity, and insertion of c-*onc* genes into normal diploid cells does not usually result in neoplastic transformation (31,126).

Modifications in the expression of viral oncogenes or cellular proto-oncogenes have been documented in a variety of virally, chemically, and spontaneously transformed tumors (146). For example, the overexpression of c-*onc*-encoded mRNA that results from the integration of viral genes in proximity to a proto-oncogene is a classic example of alteration in oncogene expression leading to transformation (46,55,106). Increased expression of oncogenes may also result from gene amplification; for example, in the *myc* gene family (3,21,26). In some cases, amplification in the expression of *myc* oncogenes has been related to the more malignant or advanced stages of neoplastic disease (14,81). This is discussed in more detail below.

Chromosome breakage and rearrangement may also result in enhanced expression of cellular oncogenes. Although the precise roles of these rearrangements in modifying oncogene expression often remain unclear, several oncogenes have been mapped at or near the sites of the chromosome alterations (122). One of the best examples of chromosomal alterations associated with aberrant expression of a cellular oncogene occurs in Burkitt's lymphoma in which a t(8;14) chromosome translocation is related to c-*myc* expression (6,139). Another is chronic myelogenous leukemia, in which a t(9;22) chromosome translocation is symptomatic of alterations in c-*abl* gene expression (22,50,56). However, it should be noted that not every tumor in a given histologic class will show these abnormal translocations; some will undergo different changes that may be unrelated to known cellular oncogenes.

Another major mechanism for altering c-*onc* genes does not necessarily involve an increase in the transcription of these genes, but it apparently alters the protein product to an "activated" form. Mutations occurring within the coding region of proto-oncogenes have been found in DNA-mediated transfection experiments, which have shown that proto-oncogenes may be activated, at least in certain cases, by a single codon base-pair change. The *ras* oncogene family, for example, can be activated by a single nucleotide change in the code for the twelfth or sixty-first amino acid of the *ras* gene product (119,136,157). Changes in *ras* genes have also been found with the transfection assay with DNA from cells transformed by chemical carcinogens. For example, chemically transformed fetal guinea pig cells show an alteration in the c-*ras* gene (134,135). Such activated oncogene products may not, however, be a common feature of tumorigenesis. Feinberg and Vogelstein (36), who examined a variety of primary human colon and lung tumors and cell lines established from these tumors, were unable to demonstrate a nucleotide change in the coding for the twelfth amino acid of the c-*ras*[H] gene, and Albino et al. (2) found inconsistent expression of activated c-*ras* genes in primary melanomas and various metastatic lesions in the same patient. Activation of oncogenes by gene mutation at specific sites apparently occurs at low frequency in human neoplasms (2,24,76).

Examination of human tumors for alterations in cellular oncogenes, such as c-*ras*, does not support the notion that oncogene mutation at specific sites is a common mechanism involved in spontaneous neoplastic transformation. Although Slamon et al. (131) found multiple alterations in oncogene expression in some primary human tumors, a number of unanswered questions remain concerning the role of such oncogenes in tumorigenesis. In most studies used to support this notion, tumor cell lines rather than primary tumors were examined for oncogene expression, and most were restricted to mRNA analyses, rather than measurements of the amounts and activities of the oncogene products.

The method of choice for detecting oncogenes from animal and human tumors has been the transfection assay (24,148). Oncogenes are usually detected by their ability to induce morphologic transformation of the mouse fibroblast line NIH/3T3. This technique has led to the identification of a series of activated cellular oncogenes in transformed animal cells and in a variety of human tumor cell lines (25,73,89,129,154). In this system, only 10% to 20% of spontaneous human tumors can be shown to have transforming activity (24,116,148). Most oncogenes discovered by this assay bleong to the *ras* group and are able to induce rapid and full tumorigenic conversion of NIH/3T3 cells. Unfortunately, NIH/3T3 cells are not ''normal''; they display a high degree of aneuploidy and high rates of spontaneous transformation. The use of such rapid one-step transformation assays with abnormal recipient cells should not therefore be confused with events that occur during the sequential changes required for spontaneous transformation. This has led some investigators to use primary embryo fibroblasts as a more ''normal'' recipient cell; but in the embryo fibroblast, oncogenes, such as those of the *ras* family, are insufficient to cause transformation, and they require the collaboration of a second oncogene, such as *myc*, to induce full tumorigenicity (76,91,124).

The choice of embryo cell lines for most transfection assays is questionable because these cells already possess some characteristics of transformation, such as high growth rates and labeling indices and certain cellular properties reminiscent of the transformed phenotype (91). In most human DNA transfection studies, the recipient cells have been nonhuman, and this could result in chromosome aberrations that are unrelated to oncogenes or to other DNA transforming sequences. To overcome this particular difficulty, Tainsky et al. (137) used PA-1 human teratocarcinoma cells that become tumorigenic (in nu/nu mice) after extensive passaging in tissue culture when a gene similar to c-ras^N is activated by point mutation. Although this system overcomes the problem of transfecting DNA across species, it still apparently requires human cells of abnormal origin that already have some, albeit apparently stable, chromosomal alterations (M. Tainsky, *personal communication*).

Another potential problem with the DNA transfection/transformation assay is that rare, susceptible cells in the population (clones) become transformed, but when expanded, these cells are usually compared with the original polyclonal cell population. The use of recently cloned cell lines for such assays should alleviate this problem, but it will not be easily eliminated. Although secondary transfection can prove that the original transfected DNA remains in the cell, this procedure probably again results in the selection of rare susceptible cells. In addition, most investigators pay scant attention to other possible changes in the transfected cell population, such as alterations in ploidy, chromosome banding, movable elements, and recombinations.

ONCOGENES AND TUMOR PROGRESSION

Alterations in oncogenes or their expression have been observed at different stages of tumor progression. For example, Abelson murine leukemia virus (AbMuLV)-transformed cells express the *abl* oncogene, and they are tumorigenic in their syngeneic hosts. After several weeks of growth *in vivo* as ascitic tumors, however, fully tumorigenic clonal cell lines derived from AbMuLV-transformed lymphomas may lose their expression of the *abl* oncogene and its encoded protein product p160 (52). We could conclude from these findings that expression of the *abl* oncogene is not required for maintenance of tumorigenicity *in vivo*. Rotter et al. (120) have examined an AbMuLV-transformed large-cell lymphoma for the expression of the *abl* oncogene and p160. Cell sublines that were originally derived for their metastatic properties by sequential *in vivo* selection for liver colonization (16) were examined for expression of *abl* and other oncogenes, but there was no difference in the expression of *abl,* its encoded product p160, or in the kinase activity of p160 within sublines of widely differing metastatic potentials (Fig. 1) (120). This system also expresses p53, a transformation-related protein. Like that of *abl*-encoded p160, the expression of p53 was similar in sublines of low or high metastatic potential (121). Transcripts of other oncogenes, including c-*myc,* were detected by mRNA probes, but again, c-*onc* gene expression and metastatic potential were not related. Although AbMuLV-transformed fibroblasts often show amplification of c-*myc* (90), these *in vitro* experiments may not be relevant to tumor progression of AbMuLV-transformed cells *in vivo*. Similarly, in the murine B16 melanoma and the UV2237 fibrosarcoma, metastatic sublines have been derived by *in vivo* selection or *in vitro* cloning. These cells express a c-*ras* oncogene, but again, there is no apparent relationship between c-*ras* transcription and metastatic potential (72). When Kris et al. (72) examined the same cells for expression of 10 other cellular oncogenes, they found the same lack of relationship between onco-

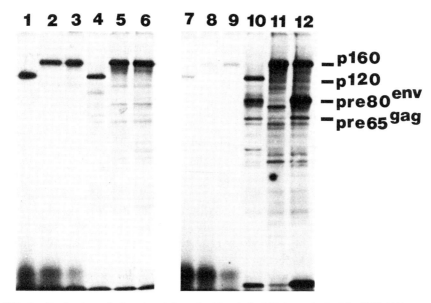

FIG. 1. Synthesis and phosphorylation of *abl*-coded p160 is equivalent in AbMuLV-transformed murine large-cell lymphoma cells of low (RAW117-P) and high (RAW117-H10) metastatic potential and in control AbLV-transformed nonmetastatic fibroblasts (2M3/M) by immunoprecipitation with two monoclonal antibodies against p160: Ab-T1 (lanes 1–6) and Ab-T2 (lanes 6–12). Lanes 1, 4, 7, 10, 2M3/M cells; lanes 2, 5, 8, 11, RAW117-P cells; lanes 3, 6, 9, 12, RAW117-H10; lanes 1–3, 7–9, γ-[^{32}P]ATP phosphorylation; lanes 4–6, 10–12, [^{35}S]methionine incorporation. (From ref. 121.)

gene expression and metastatic potential. The conclusion from these experiments is that oncogene expression and metastasis are not related. Although oncogenes may be required for the initial transforming events, their expression seems to be unrelated to the progression of tumor cells to the metastatic phenotype.

A different conclusion was reached by Vousden and Marshall (147). They examined a metastatic variant of a mouse lymphoma cell line and found that only the metastatic line contained an activated c-*ras*^{K} gene, which suggested that tumor progression in this system is related to the expression of an activated c-*onc* gene. Although their conclusions suffered from the fact that too few metastatic cell lines were examined, c-*ras*^{K} expression could be related to acquisition rather than to maintenance of the metastatic phenotype. The expression of an altered cellular oncogene could, for example, be symptomatic of other genetic events more directly related to generating cellular diversity than to malignancy (94,95).

In human tumors or cell lines derived from such tumors, the expression of c-*onc* genes has also been found to be heterogeneous and not directly related to malignancy. Recent studies showed that c-*ras* expression is variable among human melanoma cell lines originating from separate primary and secondary tumors of a single patient. Albino et al. (2) found that the DNA from four of 30 melanoma cell lines yielded transforming c-*ras*[H] genes in the NIH/3T3 transfection assay. When five cell lines isolated from the same patient's primary tumor and four metastases were examined for *ras* expression, DNA from only one line produced tumorigenic NIH/3T3 cells upon transfection, and it expressed the c-*ras*[H] oncogene and an altered p21[*ras*] protein. Albino et al. (2) found that the frequency of c-*ras* gene activation in a variety of human melanoma cell lines was approximately 13%. Along with notable heterogeneity in c-*ras* expression, these results also suggested that transforming c-*ras* genes may not be directly involved in the origin and maintenance of human melanomas but could arise as a consequence of the known genetic stability of these tumors (2).

Gallick et al. (47) directly examined the expression of the c-*ras* gene product p21[*ras*] in fresh biopsies of colorectal cancer patients. Their studies indicated that overexpression of c-*ras* genes is common (9 of 17 patients) in primary colorectal cancers of Dukes' B and C stages, compared to normal surrounding tissue. However, metastases from the more advanced Dukes' D stage (9 of 9 patients) did not show increased p21[*ras*] expression, and in fact, all metastatic lesions examined had extremely low amounts of c-*ras* expression compared with those of their primary tumors of origin. Since the antisera used to detect p21[*ras*] reacted against all known c-*ras*-related products, it is unlikely that an aberrant p21[*ras*] was expressed at high levels in the metastases. Using antibodies against p21[*ras*], Thor et al. (142) found only a few cells that stained intensely in premalignant and malignant colon tissue, a result that could reflect cellular heterogeneity of c-*ras* expression and the relative insensitivity of the immunofluorescent techniques used to localize p21[*ras*].

Data on the expression of oncogenes in human cancers and their role in progression remain unclear. Slamon et al. (131) examined oncogene expression in primary human tumors and found that many have at least one altered oncogene. Other tumors do not, however, show detectable expression of activated or elevated proto-oncogenes. Most studies on the expression of c-*onc* genes in human tumors have been limited by the examination of cell lines rather than fresh primary tumors, and when oncogene expression was noted, it was usually via mRNA analyses. Few studies have been conducted on oncogene-encoded products and their activities. Problems with sampling human tumors, such as pathologic analysis, the amount of host tissue present, and whether the patient had therapy, are usually not reported. In addition, data from metastases are often grouped with those from primary tumors.

In recent studies, amplification of c-*onc* genes was examined as a possible determinant in the progression to advanced disease states. Little et al. (81) found that amplification (20- to 76-fold) of c-*myc* in 5 of 8 human small-cell lung cancer lines correlated with the degree of malignancy. Cell variants of the usually less malignant form of small-cell lung cancer are characterized by their different enzyme profiles, the presence of differentiation antigens, faster doubling times, increased cloning efficiencies and tumorigenicities in nude mice, and resistance to X rays. All of these variant lines showed amplification in c-*myc* expression. In addition, the majority of the variant cell lines (3 of 5) examined also contained cytogenetic changes, such as a deletion in chromosome 3 and increases in double-minute chromosomes (DMs) and chromosome homogeneous staining regions (HSRs) (81). Since a c-*myc* gene has been found in association with HSRs in other human tumor cell lines [e.g., the colorectal line COLO-320 (3)], its location in an HSR could account for its amplification. However, the association of oncogene amplification with the more aggressive (more progressive?) variant lines of small-cell lung cancer does not prove that the amplified oncogene is directly involved in conferring malignant properties (as opposed to the more documentable tumorigenic properties) to the lung cancer cells. Since cell lines and not tumor specimens were used for these studies, confirmation with the use of fresh biopsied tissue samples will be required to rule out possible artifacts introduced by tissue culture.

Another report on amplification of c-*myc*^{N} in human neuroblastoma tissues also indicates a correlation with advanced disease (14). Brodeur et al. (14) examined 63 primary untreated neuroblastomas and found that in 23 cases, a c-*myc*^{N} gene had been amplified. None of five patients with stage I or II disease had amplification of c-*myc*^{N} in their tumors, whereas in 24 of 48 patients with the more advanced stage III or IV disease, significant amplification of c-*myc*^{N} was noted. In these experiments, the prevalence of c-*myc*^{N} amplification did not, however, agree with the frequency of DMs or HSRs. If amplification of c-*myc*^{N} truly represents a more malignant phenotype, it will be necessary to explain why one-half of the advanced-stage tumors did not show c-*myc*^{N} amplification.

Oncogenes and Metastasis

As described in the preceding section, changes in the expression of oncogenes in tumor cells are not always associated with expression of the metastatic phenotype. There is evidence, however, that insertion of oncogenes or related DNAs into tumor cells may result in its eventual acquisition of the metastatic phenotype. Thorgeirsson et al. (143) used the NIH/3T3 transfection system to examine the transforming and malignancy-conferring properties of DNAs from malignant human tumors. The human DNA sources were acute lymphocytic leukemia, acute myelogeneous leukemia, and T24 bladder carcinoma cells bearing activated c-*ras* oncogenes. Some 2 to 3 weeks after 3T3 cell transfection, representative foci were picked for a second round of DNA transfection. All secondary transfectants examined were tumorigenic in nude mice and formed fibrosarcomas that contained activated c-*ras*^{N} or c-*ras*^{H} genes. Subcutaneous injection of the NIH/3T3 cells containing activated c-*ras*^{H} (but not cells containing activated c-*ras*^{N}) oncogenes produced spontaneous metastases within 4 weeks. One of the 3T3 transformants obtained from T24 DNA transfection was examined for such metastasis-associated properties as type IV collagenase activity and amnion basement membrane invasion capacity, and it was found to possess these two characteristics that are indicative of metastatic cells (92,93). Host effector mechanisms, such as natural killer- and macrophage-mediated cytotoxicity, were similar among the transfectants and parental 3T3 cells, indicating that the transfected cells were not metastatic because of acquired resistance to host immune defenses. The T24-transfected metastatic 3T3 cells and cells from a solitary lung metastasis showed a twofold increase in c-ras^N expression, but more recent data (144) indicate wide variation in c-ras expression in metastatic cell foci and no apparent relationship in the expression of this onco-gene and metastatic properties. In many of the cell lines established from sponta-neous metastases of c-ras^H-transfected NIH/3T3 cells, the expression of c-ras^H was at the same level or lower than in the original tumors. The authors speculate that DNA transfection could accelerate the rate of tumor progression rather than di-rectly confer metastatic properties, a proposal advanced previously to account for the absence of a correlation between oncogene expression and metastatic proper-ties (94,95). Future efforts in this area should concentrate on the specific genome alterations produced by DNA transfection, including chromosomal changes and genetic alterations in genes unrelated to c-onc genes.

Using DNA isolated from the human EJ bladder carcinoma cell line, Bernstein and Weinberg (9) transfected NIH/3T3 cells and isolated c-ras^H-expressing trans-formants that produced nonmetastatic fibrosarcomas in immunocompetent alloge-neic mice. These same c-ras^H-transfected 3T3 cells formed metastases in nu/nu nude mice, indicating that immunologic barriers may have prevented metastasis in the allogeneic mice and that further changes are necessary to generate the meta-static phenotype. When the NIH/3T3 cells were transfected with control DNA, only 1 of 38 mice developed metastases 6 weeks after subcutaneous injection. In contrast, intravenous injection of mice resulted in experimental lung metastases in 4 of 4 animals. When the c-ras^H-transfected 3T3 cells were transfected again with DNAs from a variety of human tumor cell lines, plus a selectable marker, and the cell colonies were grown in the presence of a selecting antibiotic, tumorigenic cell colonies were obtained, but only one of these formed a metastasis. This indicated that most 3T3 transfectants harboring DNA from malignant cells are not meta-static; but the authors explained this in terms of low gene dosage effects in the primary transfection. DNA was prepared from cells of the one metastasis, and this was used to retransfect the c-ras^H-transformed cells, whereupon most animals in-jected subcutaneously with the secondary 3T3 transfectants displayed fibrosarcoma metastases. The DNA of tertiary transfectants contained the c-ras^H oncogene origi-nally transfected into the 3T3 cells, but the additional transfected human DNA segment was not the ras^K, ras^N, or myc oncogene. Although the transfected human DNA segment was not identified as a distinct human gene, the result indicated that further changes may be necessary for transformed cells to become metastatic in allogeneic hosts.

A major problem in the experimental approaches using transfection is that ge-netic manipulation itself may initiate genetic instability that may eventually result in acquisition of the metastatic phenotype (94,95). When Grieg et al. (49) exam-ined c-ras^H-1-gene transfected NIH/3T3 cells for their tumorigenic and metastatic properties, they found that the c-ras oncogene accelerated the tumorigenic proper-ties and enhanced the metastatic potential of the 3T3 cells. Yet, they also found that high numbers of untransfected NIH/3T3 cells were tumorigenic and metastatic some 20 weeks after injection into nude mice. Grieg et al. (49) indicated that caution should be used in interpreting the results of transfection experiments in which dubious "preneoplastic" cell lines, such as NIH/3T3 fibroblasts, are used as recipients. Similar results were obtained by Eccles et al. (32) when they transfected the plasmid pSV2Neo or the c-*ras*^{H}-1-gene from human T24 bladder carcinoma cells in a pSV2Neo vector into essentially nonmetastatic mouse mammary carcinoma cells. The c-*ras*^{H}-1 transfected cells grew more rapidly at subcutaneous sites, formed more spontaneous metastases, and killed recipient mice faster than did the control pSV2Neo-transfected cells. However, the pSV2Neo-transfected cells, in turn, were more malignant than the nonmetastatic parental mammary tumor cells and formed spontaneous metastases in a variety of organs. One of the pSV2Neo-transfected cell lines killed animals almost as fast as one of the c-*ras*^{H}-1-transfected lines, which suggested that genome alterations caused by transfection resulted in cellular instability and progression of the transfected cells to a more malignant phenotype.

Gene Expression in Metastatic Cells

Differential gene expression has been studied in a variety of developmental and neoplastic systems by differential hybridization of mRNAs using clonal libraries of expressed gene sequences. Most researchers have constructed cDNA libraries from poly(A$^+$) RNA of one or two cell populations. Using [^{32}P]cDNA synthesized from the different poly(A$^+$) RNA of two cell types, the sequences in these libraries can be probed to identify specific genes that are expressed in relatively higher or lower amounts in the two cell populations (51). For example, Shiosaka and Saunders (130) compared gene expression in chronic lymphocytic leukemia with that of various hematopoietic cells and found a series of genes that were differentially expressed in human neoplastic leukocytes. In studies of low-metastatic and *in vivo*-selected high-metastatic AbMuLV-transformed large-cell lymphomas, differential gene expression was correlated with malignancy (99). In this case, a highly metastatic liver-colonizing lymphoma subline showed loss of expression of viral-specific mRNA concomitant with loss of viral gene encoded gp70, p30, and p15 (118), but no difference in the expression of *abl* or other oncogenes (120). Subtracting the virally related sequences demonstrated that only a few nonviral genes were differentially expressed in the metastatic cells. Since oncogene expression was the same as in the highly metastatic cells, these data showed that malignancy was not related to oncogene amplification or increased expression. This is not surprising, since oncogene-encoded products seem to be more related to growth regulation than to malignancy (62,146). In similar studies, Augenlicht et al. (4) used a cDNA library prepared from poly(A$^+$)RNA of human colon carcinoma cells to examine differential gene expression. Using cDNA probes prepared from normal flat mucosa, premalignant adenoma, and frank carcinoma, these authors identified a number of gene sequences that are characteristic of normal, benign, and malignant cells.

Antigen loss is one mechanism that can affect the survival and malignant properties of antigenic tumor cells in immunocompetent hosts (92,97). During tumor progression, malignant cells undoubtedly undergo selection by host effector mechanisms leading to, in many cases, selection of tumor cells with decreased immunogenicities and increased resistance to host effector mechanisms. When highly metastatic cells were examined for expression of strong cell surface antigens, they were often found to express lower amounts than their nonmetastatic or low-metastatic counterparts (29,118). Using the Lewis lung carcinoma metastatic model, differences were also noted in multiple histocompatibility complex (MHC) antigen expression (33). The ratio of $H\text{-}2K^b/H\text{-}2D^b$ expression in this system appears to be indicative of the metastatic phenotype: the lower the ratio, the more the cells expressed the metastatic phenotype. The possible role of MHC antigen loss in generating the metastatic phenotype has been studied in the B16 melanoma system (138). The spontaneously metastatic B16-BL6 cell line ($H\text{-}2^b$) was transfected with a gene coding for the $H\text{-}2D^d$ antigen, and the resulting $H\text{-}2^d$-expressing cells were injected into syngeneic nonimmune mice or syngeneic mice immunized against $H\text{-}2^d$ antigens. Primary subcutaneous tumor growth was affected only in the immunized animals, but host survival was prolonged in both groups. When the transfected tumor cells were isolated from lung metastases or from progressively growing subcutaneous tumors in immunized animals and examined for H-2 expression, they showed partial or complete loss of the transfected $H\text{-}2D^d$ plasmid, indicating that the host was probably responsible for selection of antigen-loss highly malignant cell variants (138).

GENOMIC INSTABILITY AND PROGRESSION

The concept of tumor progression advanced by Foulds (43) and Nowell (100) evokes the concept that increasing numbers of genetic alterations (''genetic instability'') are generated by random somatic mutational events and, furthermore, that these genetic changes in concert with host selection allow the eventual emergence of tumor cell subpopulations that have altered malignant and other phenotypic properties (Fig. 2). It is thought that new tumor cell subpopulations that have undergone rapid diversification and become dominant should display enhanced genetic instability and acquire those properties most favorable to their survival and growth in the face of host selection pressures.

The hypothesis that neoplasms undergoing progression to the malignant phenotype possess enhanced genetic instability has gained support from cytogenetic and genetic experiments. Comparisons of gross chromosomal alterations, mitotic errors, and rates of spontaneous mutations in highly malignant cells compared with those in benign or less malignant cells indicates that malignancy is associated with gross genomic instability (101,155). In advanced malignancies, chromosomal abnormalities or alterations in the numbers, morphologies, and banding patterns of specific chromosomes become progressively more pronounced as the malignant tu-

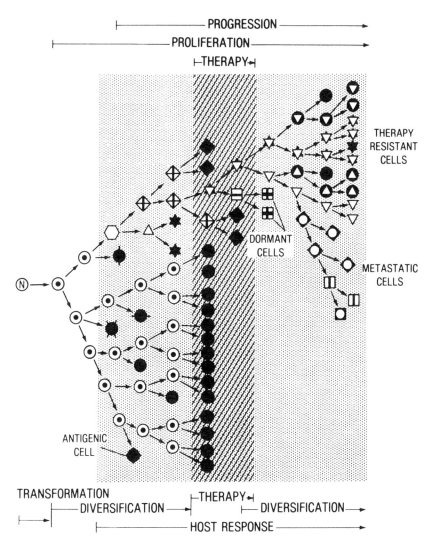

FIG. 2. Tumor phenotypic diversification and progression and the effect of antitumor therapy. Transformation of a normal cell (N) to a tumor cell can lead to cellular diversification in malignant neoplasms. Some of these variant tumor cells die *(solid symbols)* due to lethal mutations or host responses, or they fail to grow and become dormant, whereas other tumor cells become more competitive and malignant as they undergo phenotypic diversification. Cytotoxic therapy results in the death of most tumor cells *(solid symbols)* and restriction of phenotypic diversity; however, some malignant cells escape randomly or due to therapeutic resistance and continue to diversify phenotypically. Eventually, a malignant subpopulation arises that possesses the correct phenotypic properties for metastasis. (From ref. 94.)

mor progresses (102). As malignant cells evolve, such chromosomal abnormalities may increase in frequency, reflecting the appearance and evolution of a specific cell clone with further alterations (101).

Most of the data on chromosomal changes associated with tumor progression have been derived from studies of human leukemias and lymphomas, although some data gathered from solid tumors support this hypothesis. In the early indolent stage of progressive, chronic granulocytic leukemia, the cells of most patients typically show only the appearance of a minute chromosome, Ph^1, whereas the terminal accelerated phase of the disease often results from the outgrowth of one or more subclones having additional karyotypic changes, such as an extra chromosome 8 and a 9;22 translocation (122). In Burkitt's lymphoma, almost all tumors have been found to contain characteristic translocations that juxtapose c-*myc* to one of three immunoglobulin loci and result in activation of the c-*myc* oncogene (68). Chromosome deletions and inversions may affect gene expression similarly. In Abelson virus-producing murine plasmacytomas, interstitial deletions of band D of chromosome 15 correlate with enhanced expression of the c-*myc* oncogene, which has been localized near or at this chromosome site (150).

Chromosomal changes are apparent also during progression of malignant animal tumors. In Rous sarcoma virus-transformed fibroblasts, consistent chromosomal changes were associated with tumor progression: first, the appearance of an extra chromosome 7, followed by the acquisition of an additional chromosome 13, and finally an extra chromosome 12 (79). A number of chromosome markers were identified in rat tumor cell clones isolated from malignant mammary tumors growing at primary, regional lymph node, and lung metastatic sites (107). In these studies, the most metastatic cell clones were found to possess a particular set of Giemsa-stained chromosome markers at high frequencies, and they had other markers in common with the primary and lymph node tumors.

Human malignant melanomas have been studied by examining both primary and secondary lesions (60,102). In all cases so far examined, the primary tumor is characterized by a cytogenetically abnormal cell, and the tumor's metastases showed the same cytogenetic alterations in addition to other changes. Moreover, regional variability was found in the same primary melanoma. Cells from the deeply invasive portions (vertical growth phase) of tumors showed karyotypic changes more like those of the metastases than the primary tumor areas of lower invasiveness (radial growth phase). Specifically, the cells from the vertical growth phase and metastases showed alterations involving chromosomes 1 and 6, and the metastatic cells contained additional copies of chromosome 7. Although only limited cytogenetic data are available, human primary neuroblastomas and their metastases were also shown to share marker chromosomes. In addition, the metastases possessed further alterations, such as additional chromosomes and new chromosome markers (35).

As mentioned above, cellular oncogenes have been mapped in at least some malignancies at or near the translocation breakpoints in altered chromosomes. For example, many animal and human B-cell tumor lines possess chromosome translocations in the area of the c-*myc* gene (68). Burkitt's lymphomas harboring the t(8;14) chromosome translocation are associated with aberrant expression of the c-*myc* oncogene (34,139), and chronic myelogenous leukemias possessing a t(9;22) alteration in the area of the c-*abl* gene often show c-*abl* amplification (22,56).

In many human malignancies, increases in chromosome number are often related to advanced stages of the disease and poor prognosis (5,155). For example, progression to metastatic disease is frequently associated with hyperdiploidy (74,141); however, it is more likely that specific chromosomal changes will prove to be more important in phenotypic diversity and progression that generalized increases in cell ploidy (95).

Genetic instability of highly malignant tumors has been estimated in animal metastatic systems by determining the spontaneous rates of gene mutation. Cifone and Fidler (20) examined the rates of spontaneous mutation by using several drug-resistant markers in murine melanoma and fibrosarcoma cells of differing metastatic potentials. Selected cell sublines and clones of high metastatic potential, for example, had about six- to seven-fold higher rates of spontaneous mutation to drug resistance than their less metastatic or benign counterparts.

There exist a number of different possible mechanisms for generating genotypic instability (19,101). These are thought to include: inherited defects in DNA repair or maintenance genes; acquired defects in specialized genes, such as "mutator" genes or genes involved in synthesizing DNA; chromosomal alterations, such as aneuploidy, transpositions, abnormal sister-chromatidic changes, HSRs, and DMs; integrated virus sequences or v-*onc* genes; mutagenic agents, such as radiation or chemotherapeutic drugs; and microenvironmental alterations, such as nutritional differences and growth and differentiation modulators (94,95,101). These potential mechanisms may not produce the same end results; they may be more common in some tumor types and not occur at all in others.

PHENOTYPIC INSTABILITY AND TUMOR PROGRESSION

Although the genesis of tumor phenotypic diversification and progression undoubtedly revolves around genotypic instability and its manifestations, mechanisms other than genotypic instability and host selection are necessary to explain the rates of neoplastic progression and tumor diversification seen in many systems. Genotypic instability alone cannot explain the extremely high rates of tumor cell phenotypic variation that are often found. For example, the highest known rates of spontaneous gene mutation, such as the 7×10^{-5}/cell/generation found by Cifone and Fidler (20), are orders of magnitude lower than the rates of phenotypic variation measured by biological, biochemical, and immunological changes in tumor cells. One can argue that phenotypic changes may be based on a series of quantitative rather than qualitative changes, and it is unlikely that these could be found with the techniques discussed above. Alternatively, mutations or rearrangements could occur at regulatory gene sites. That modifications in regulatory genes occur in malignant cells is not unreasonable, since most changes in gene products associated with the malignant phenotype appear to be quantitative (93,95).

The rates of phenotypic diversification have been estimated for a number of human and animal tumors, and in some cases these have been compared to their normal cell counterparts. For example, Peterson et al. (110) estimated the rates of quantitative variation in the single-cell expression of a $M_r \sim 400,00$ surface glycoprotein on normal breast epithelial cells and on breast carcinoma cells. The rate of appearance of significant quantitative cell variants in the cell population was about six times higher (mean, $\sim 2.2 \times 10^{-2}$/cell/generation) in malignant breast cancer cells than in normal breast epithelial cells (mean, $\sim 0.36 \times 10^{-2}$/cell/generation). Rapid rates of phenotypic diversification are not unusual in malignant neoplasms and have been observed in several tumor systems by cell cloning (13,53, 61,80,132,152,153).

The rates of phenotypic change in tumor cell populations do not seem to be constant and can be modulated by interactions between cell subpopulations in the tumor. Poste et al. (113) found that by mixing several clonal populations of B16 melanoma, they could "stabilize" the cell clones and reduce their normally rapid rates of metastatic phenotypic diversification. Not all properties were modified by these cellular interactions. In their studies, cells were selected repeatedly for drug-resistant phenotypes, and the drug-resistant properties of the cell clones appeared to be stable. In the B16 melanoma system, Fidler and Nicolson (42) had found that although polyclonal B16 melanoma cell populations were relatively stable during long-term culture, cell clones generated from these populations were highly unstable. In highly metastatic B16 cells, such as the brain-colonizing sublines selected *in vivo* for brain metastasis, clonal derivatives were unstable during *in vivo* propagation (86). Mixing three of the separately grown B16 cell clones together just before injection into animals did not stabilize their brain-colonization properties. When these same cell clones were allowed to grow together as a triclonal mixture, however, phenotypic stabilization occurred, and their metastatic and cell surface properties were maintained (86). The possible mechanism of polyclonal stabilization of phenotypic diversification of malignant cells has remained elusive, although some evidence suggests that molecular signals may be passed from some cell clones to others in the polyclonal population (115).

Modifications in the phenotypic stability of tumor cells can also occur *in vivo* by the fusion of neoplastic with normal cells to form cell hybrids (48). Modifications in phenotypic properties, as well as tumor cell ploidy, could be accounted for in some systems by cell fusion. It is now known that fusion of nonmetastatic cells to normal cells can result in the generation of a metastatic heterokaryon. De-Baetselier et al. (28) found that fusion of nonmetastatic mouse plasmacytoma cells with normal B cells can result in hybrids that are highly metastatic to liver and spleen. Lagarde et al. (75) have proposed that the emergence of highly metastatic variant cells from a population of less metastatic lectin-resistant cells during growth *in vivo* is consistent with hybridization of a nonmetastatic cell with a normal host cell (in this case, probably a monocyte), and this results in the eventual progression and domination of a hyperdiploid metastatic cell. Progression in this system was associated with an initial increase in cell ploidy, followed by extensive chromosome segregation. The role of specific chromosomal and possible mutational changes in this process, however, has not yet been discerned.

Specific tumor cell subpopulations, such as drug-resistant variants, can emerge during cancer therapy. For example, it is well known that differential therapeutic responses often exist between primary tumors and their metastases (45,82,145). As discussed above, the presence of specific tumor cell subpopulations in the polyclonal tumor could restrict the rate at which variant cells are generated (96,112). Mammary tumor cell subpopulations can regulate one another's growth, which results in stabilizing the tumor cell subpopulation as a whole and in restricting phenotypic diversity (84,85). When Poste et al. (113) examined the effects of cytotoxic drugs on the phenotypic diversity of B16 melanoma cells, they found that cytotoxic drugs can deplete the polyclonal melanoma cell population of drug-sensitive cells to yield surviving cell clones that are highly unstable phenotypically; but the unstable clones quickly generated a new panel of cell subpopulations with differing metastatic and other properties. This new panel of cells seemed to evolve into a mixed population, which was apparently stabilized by polyconal interactions, since it did not continue to generate cell variants at the same rate. These data indicate that cellular interactions within at least some tumors may be important in stabilizing phenotypic properties and in controlling the rate at which variant cells emerge within the population.

Epigenetic Effects

Since phenotypic diversification of malignant tumors cannot be explained easily by considering solely rates of genetic mutation and host selection, additional proposals have been advanced involving modifications in regulatory genes, rapid alterations in gene or chromosome arrangements (for example, recombination), or integration of extrachromosomal DNA sequences (for example, v-*onc* genes). These changes may amplify or modulate the normal controls that determine phenotype stability. An alternative nongenetic explanation for the higher rates of phenotypic instability seen in malignant neoplasms is the proposal that epigenetic mechanisms result in nonmutational DNA modifications, which in turn alter gene regulation and expression (44,65). Epigenetic modifications of genomic DNA, such as hypomethylation, can result in alterations of gene expression without modifying gene sequences. In addition, such epigenetic modifications may persist for several generations before reverting slowly to the previous state.

DNA methylation is one of the more interesting cellular mechanisms that is assumed to be epigenetic. It is well known that transcription can be altered by the methylation of cytosine residues, resulting in hypomethylation and activation of specific genes (63,117). Using the nucleoside analog 5-aza-cytidine, Jones and Taylor (63) demonstrated that hypomethylation may lead to short-term heritable phenotypic changes in cells. In these experiments, 5-aza-cytidine produced relatively stable modifications in cells without changing gene sequences. The tumorigenic and metastatic phenotypes of murine cell lines have been altered by use of 5-aza-cytidine (65). Drug treatment caused rapid phenotypic changes, such as loss of tumorigenicity in up to 80% of tumor cell clones tested. These phenotypic changes were eventually lost, however, as the cell clones reverted to their original phenotypes. Kerbel et al. (65) also induced the metastatic phenotype at high rates in certain nonmetastatic cell clones by 5-aza-cytidine treatment. Feinberg and Vogelstein (36) in examining DNA methylation patterns in primary tumors and metastases showed that selected genes in metastases from colon carcinoma contained less methylated DNA than the primary tumors of the same patient. Although it has been argued that such drugs as 5-aza-cytidine are nonmutagenic, under certain conditions they might cause genetic rather than epigenetic changes.

A variety of other nongenetic processes could be important in regulating gene expression and the rates at which gene products are formed (15,27); however, the role of these postgenetic processes in regulating phenotypic diversification remains unknown.

Microenvironmental Effects

Cells within a tumor are influenced by neighboring cells. Such influence also extends to the tumor's microenvironment. Since individual neoplastic cells experience unique microenvironments because of variability in concentrations of nutrients, oxygen, growth hormones, enzymes, ions, as well as cellular inducers, modulators, and other regulatory molecules, the action of these external conditions and agents on individual tumor cells may in part determine their phenotypic stabilities (94,95).

One of the more important microenvironmental factors in the growth and differentiation of tumor cells is their interaction with the extracellular matrix or stromal components. These interactions can result in the turning on of specific gene programs (11). Extracellular matrix components important in such interactions include basal laminae or basement membranes; tissue matrix and extracellular elements synthesized by parenchymal cells and endothelial cells, and by fibroblasts, mesothelial cells, and other cell types capable of nonimmune "host reactions" involving stromal components. The extracellular matrix environments around cells and tissues are important in maintaining states of proliferation and differentiation. Although the responses to such interactions are often modified in neoplastic cells, they are believed to be at least partially capable of responding to their microenvironments.

In addition to insoluble matrices that signal and regulate cells, soluble molecules, such as differentiation inducers and modulators, hormones and growth factors, are involved in controlling normal cellular growth and differentiation. That tumor cells can be induced to respond to such environmental signals, which results in reversion of the malignant phenotype to a normal or benign phenotype, has been shown by Sachs (125). For example, phenotypic reversion to a more "normal" phenotype has been accomplished in myeloid leukemia cells using macrophage and granulocyte inducer or colony-stimulating factors (77,83). Soluble molecules may be responsible, in part, for mediating the phenotypic changes seen in teratocarcinoma cells when they are implanted in normal blastocysts, where they develop into phenotypically normal cells and tissues (87,111). The microenvironment of the normal blastocyst is thought to modulate the implanted malignant cells. Not all malignant cells placed into the blastocyst cavity develop normally, however, which indicates that tumor cells vary in their abilities to respond to microenvironmental signals (111).

Tumors often show extensive infiltration by such host cells as lymphocytes, granulocytes, and macrophages, among others. When such cells are in close proximity to the tumor cells, they may have profound effects on tumor cell growth and phenotypic diversification. Normal host cells such as macrophages and granulocytes may release mutagenic substances like H_2O_2 that can affect spontaneous rates of mutation (58). Thus, in addition to selection processes based on mechanisms that result in cytolysis and/or cytostasis, surviving tumor cells may be exposed to a microenvironment conducive to spontaneous gene mutation.

FINAL COMMENTS

The emergence of diversified cell subpopulations in malignant tumors, some of which are characterized by their abilities to invade, disseminate, implant, survive, and grow at secondary sites, results eventually in tumor progression. Although this process is believed to occur in a stepwise fashion, it is likely a continuium with rapidly reversible steps (80) and major forward events, such as gross chromosomal changes and gene mutations, that are less reversible. These major events could be critical in the evolution of the metastatic phenotype, since it depends on so many cellular properties (92,93).

The close similarity of many malignant cell properties to those involved in normal cell proliferation, differentiation, and development is no accident (123). The genes that control or code for many of these same cellular properties are probably the genes that have been mistermed "metastasis genes." In normal cells these genes are usually under very strict controls, and it is probably the controlling mechanisms (possibly similar to cancer "suppressor" genes) that become inevitably compromised. This is also seen in laboratory situations in which "strong" (dominant acting) v-*onc* genes can misappropriate cellular growth controls and possibly enhance cellular instability.

Cellular diversification is itself a normal process required for development and differentiation (123). Even in normal adult organisms, diversification mechanisms exist for specialized purposes; for example, the somatic diversification of lymphocyte stem cells results in the formation of mature antibody-producing B cells. It is extremely interesting that cellular oncogenes seem to be present in the same gene regions that are involved in at least some diversification processes. Could it be that insertion, recombination, or modification of oncogenes or other genes near developmentally regulated gene families leads to stimulation or modification of diversification mechanisms (94,95)? This notion is probably too simplistic; but, it seems to be supported by data indicating that transfection of control genes, such as *Neo*, can also to a certain degree stimulate cellular diversification and evolution of metastatic variants. The problem with this and other proposals is that we know so little about the cellular changes that are involved in generating and maintaining cellular diversification and the metastatic phenotype.

REFERENCES

1. Adams, J.M, Gerondakis, S., Webb, E., Corcoran, L.M., and Cory, S. (1983): Cellular *myc* oncogene is altered by chromosome translocation in murine plasmacytomas is rearranged similarly in human Burkitt lymphomas. *Proc. Natl. Acad. Sci. U.S.A.,* 80:1982–1986.
2. Albino, A.P., LeStrange, R., Oliff, A.I., Furth, M.E., and Old, L.J. (1984): Transforming *ras* genes from human melanoma: A manifestation of tumour heterogeneity? *Nature,* 308:69–72.
3. Alitalo, K., Schwab, M., Lin, C.C., Varmus, H.E., and Bishop, J.M. (1983): Homogenously staining chromosomal regions contain amplified copies of an abundantly expressed cellular oncogene (c-*myc*) in malignant neuroendocrine cells from a human colon carcinoma. *Proc. Natl. Acad. Sci. U.S.A.,* 80:1707–1711.
4. Augenlicht, L., Wahrman, M., Halsey, H., Kenna, M., Anderson, L., Taylor, J., and Lipkin, M. (1985): Expression of cDNA clones in human colon cancer [Abstract]. *Proc. Assoc. Cancer Res.,* 26:6.
5. Barlogie, B., Johnston, D.A., and Smallwood, l. (1982): Prognostic implications of ploidy and proliferative activity in human solid tumors. *Cancer Genet. Cytogenet.,* 6:17–28.
6. Battey, J., Moulding, C., Taub, R., Murphy, W., Stewart, T., Potter, H., Lenoir, G., and Leder, P. (1983): The human c-*myc* oncogene: Structural consequences of translocation into the IgH locus in Burkitt lymphoma. *Cell,* 34:779–787.
7. Benedict, W.F., Murphree, A.L., Banerjee, A., Spina, C.A., Sparkes, M.C., and Sparkes, R.S. (1983): Patient with 13 chromosome deletion: Evidence that the retinoblastoma gene is a recessive cancer gene. *Science,* 219:973–974.
8. Benedict, W.F., Weissman, B.E., Mark, C., and Stanbridge, E.J. (1984): Tumorigenicity of human HT1080 fibrosarcoma × normal fibroblast hybrids: Chromosome dosage dependency. *Cancer Res.,* 44:3471–3479.
9. Bernstein, S.C., and Weinberg, R.A. (1985): Expression of the metastatic phenotype in cells transfected with human metastatic tumor DNA. *Proc. Natl. Acad. Sci. U.S.A.,* 82:1726–1730.
10. Bishop, J.M. (1983): Cellular oncogenes and retroviruses. *Annu. Rev. Biochem.,* 52:301–354.
11. Bissel, M.J., Hall, H.G., and Parry, G. (1983): How does the extracellular matrix direct gene expression? *J. Theor. Biol.,* 99:31–68.
12. Blanchard, J.M., Piechaczyk, M., Dani, C., Chambard, J.C., Franchi, A., Pouyssegur, J., and Jeanteur, P. (1985): c-*Myc* gene is transcribed at high rate in G_0-arrested fibroblasts and is post-transcriptionally regulated in response to growth factors. *Nature,* 317:443–445.
13. Bosslet, K., and Schirrmacher, V. (1982): High-frequency generation of new immunoresistant tumor variants during metastasis of a clone murine tumor line (ESb). *Int. J. Cancer,* 29:195–202.
14. Brodeur, G., Seeger, C., Schwab, M., Varmus, H.E., and Bishop, J.M. (1984): Amplification of N-*myc* in untreated human neuroblastomas correlates with advanced disease stage. *Science,* 224:1121–1124.
15. Brown, D.D. (1981): Gene expression in eukaryotes. *Science,* 211:667–674.
16. Brunson, K.W., and Nicolson, G.L. (1978): Selection and biologic properties of malignant variants of a murine lymphoma. *J. Natl. Cancer Inst.,* 61:1499–1503.
17. Cairns, J. (1981): The origin of human cancers. *Nature,* 289:353–357.
18. Chaganti, R.S.K. (1983): The significance of chromosome change to neoplastic development. In: *Chromosome Mutation and Neoplasia,* edited by J. German, pp. 359–396, Alan R. Liss, Inc., New York.

19. Chorazy, M. (1985): Sequence rearrangements and genome instability. *J. Cancer Res. Clin. Oncol.,* 109:159–172.

20. Cifone, M.A., and Fidler, I.J. (1981): Increasing metastatic potential is associated with increasing genetic instability of clones isolated from murine neoplasms. *Proc. Natl. Acad. Sci. U.S.A.,* 78:6949–6952.

21. Collins, S.J., and Groudine, M. (1982): Amplification of endogenous *myc*-related DNA sequences in a human myeloid leukaemia cell line. *Nature,* 298:679–681.

22. Collins, S.J., and Groudine, M. (1983): Rearrangement and amplification of c-*abl* sequences in the human chronic myelogenous leukaemia cell line K-562. *Proc. Natl. Acad. Sci. U.S.A.,* 80:4813–4817.

23. Collins, S.J., Kubonishi, I., Miyoshi, I., and Groudine, M. (1984): Altered transcription of the c-*abl* oncogene in K-562 and other chronic myelogenous leukaemia cells. *Science,* 225:72–74.

24. Cooper, G.M. (1982): Cellular transforming genes. *Science,* 217:801–806.

25. Cooper, G.M., Okenquist, S., and Silverman, L. (1980): Transforming activity of DNA of chemically transformed and normal cells. *Nature,* 284:418–421.

26. Dalla-Favera, R., Wong-Stall, F., and Gallo, R.C. (1982): Onc-gene amplication in promyelocytic leukaemia cell lines HL-60 and primary leukaemic cells of the same patient. *Nature.* 298:61–63.

27. Darnell, J.E., Jr. (1982): Variety in the level of gene control in eukaryotic cells. *Nature,* 297:365–371.

28. DeBaetselier, P., Gorelik, E., Eshhar, Z., Ron, Y., Katzav, S., Feldman, M., and Segal, S. (1981): Metastatic properties conferred on nonmetastatic tumors by hybridization of spleen α-lymphocytes with plasmocytoma cells. *J. Natl. Cancer Inst.,* 67:1079–1087.

29. Dennis, J., Donaghue, T., Florian, M., and Kerbel, R.S. (1981): Apparent reversion of stable *in vitro* genetic markers detected in tumour cells from spontaneous metastases. *Nature,* 292:242–245.

30. Doolittle, R.F., Hunkapiller, M.W., Hood, L.E., DeVare, S.G., Robbins, K.C., Aaronson, S.A., and Antoniades, H.N. (1983): Simian sarcoma virus *onc* gene, v-*sis*, is derived from the gene (or genes) encoding a platelet-derived growth factor. *Science,* 221:275–276.

31. Duesberg, P.H. (1985): Activated proto-onc genes: Sufficient or necessary for cancer? *Science,* 228:669–677.

32. Eccles, S.A., Marshall, C.J., Vousden, K., and Purvies, H.P. (1985): Enhanced spontaneous metastatic capacity of mammary carcinoma cells transfected with H-*ras*. In: *Treatment of Metastasis: Problems and Prospects,* edited by K. Hellman, and S.A. Eccles, pp. 385–388, Taylor and Francis, London.

33. Eisenbach, L., Segal, S., and Feldman, M. (1983): MHC inbalance and metastatic spread in Lewis lung carcinoma clones. *Int. J. Cancer,* 32:113–120.

34. Erikson, J., ar-Rushdi, A., Drowinga, H.L., Nowell, P.C., and Croce, C.M. (1983): Transcriptional activation of the translocated c-*myc* oncogene in Burkitt's lymphoma. *Proc. Natl. Acad. Sci. U.S.A.,* 80:820–824.

35. Feder, M.K., and Gilbert, F. (1983): Clonal evolution in a human neuroblastoma. *J. Natl. Cancer Inst.,* 70:1051–1056.

36. Feinberg, A., and Vogelstein, B. (1983): Hypomethylation distinguishes genes of some human cancers from their normal counterparts. *Nature* 301:89–92.

37. Feinberg, A.P., Vogelstein, B., Droller, M.J., Baylin, S.B., and Nelkin, B.D. (1983): Mutation affecting the twelfth amino acid of the c-Ha-*ras* oncogene product occurs infrequently in human cancer. *Science,* 220:1175–1177.

38. Fialkow, P.J. (1979): Clonal origin of human tumors. *Annu. Rev. Med.,* 30:135–176.

39. Fialkow, P.J., Gartler, S.M., and Yoshida, A. (1967): Clonal origin of chronic myelocytic leukemia in man. *Proc. Natl. Acad. Sci. U.S.A.,* 58:1468–1471.

40. Fidler, I.J., and Hart, I.R. (1982): Biological diversity in metastatic neoplasms origins and implications. *Science,* 217:998–1003.

41. Fidler, I.J., Gerstein, D.M., and Hart, I.R. (1978): The biology of cancer invasion and metastasis. *Adv. Cancer Res.,* 28:149–250.

42. Fidler, I.J., and Nicolson, G.L. (1981): Immunobiology of experimental metastatic melanoma. *Cancer Biol. Rev.,* 2:171–234.

43. Foulds, L., ed. (1975): *Neoplastic Development.* Academic Press, New York.

44. Frost, P., and Kerbel, R.S. (1983): On a possible epigenetic mechanism(s) of tumor cell heterogeneity. *Cancer Metastasis Rev.,* 2:375–378.

45. Fugmann, R.A., Anderson, J.C., Stolf, R.L., and Martin, D.S. (1977): Comparison of adjuvant chemotherapeutic activity against primary and metastatic spontaneous murine tumors. *Cancer Res.*, 57:496–500.
46. Fung, Y.K.T., Lewis, W.G., Kung, H.J., and Crittenden, L.B. (1983): Activation of the cellular oncogene c-*erb*B by LTR insertion: Molecular basis for induction of erythroblastosis by avian leukosis virus. *Cell*, 33:357–368.
47. Gallick, G.E., Kurzrock, R., Kloetzer, W.S., Arlinghaus, R.B., and Gutterman, J.U. (1985): Expression of the p21 *ras* gene products in fresh primary and metastatic human colorectal tumors. *Proc. Natl. Acad. Sci. U.S.A.*, 82:1795–1799.
48. Goldenberg, D.M., Pavia, R.A., and Tsao, M.C. (1974): *In vivo* hybridization of human tumor and normal hamster cells. *Nature*, 250:649–651.
49. Greig, R.G., Koestler, T.P., Trainer, D.L., Corwin, S.P., Miles, L., Kline, T., Sweet, R., Yokoyama, S., and Poste, G. (1985): Tumorigenic and metastatic properties of "normal" and *ras*-transfected NIH/3T3 cells. *Proc. Natl. Acad. Sci. U.S.A.*, 82:3698–3701.
50. Groffen, J., Stephenson, J.R., Heisterkamp, N., deKlein, A., Bartram, C.R., and Grosveld, G. (1984): Philadelphia chromosomal breakpoints are clustered within a limited region, *bcr*, on chromosome 22. *Cell*, 36:93–99.
51. Grunstein, M., and Hogness, D.S. (1975): Colony hybridization: A method for the isolation of cloned DNAs that contain a specific gene. *Proc. Natl. Acad. Sci. U.S.A.*, 72:3961–3965.
52. Grunwald, D.J., Dale, B., Dudley, J., Lamph, W., Sugden, B., Ozanne, B., and Kisser, R. (1982): Loss of viral gene expression and retention of tumorigenicity by Abelson lymphoma cells. *J. Virol.*, 43:92–103.
53. Harris, J.F., Chambers, A.F., Hill, R.P., and Ling, V. (1982): Metastatic variants are generated spontaneously at a high rate in mouse KHT tumor. *Proc. Natl. Acad. Sci. U.S.A.*, 79:5547–5551.
54. Hart, I.R., and Fidler, I.J. (1981): The implications of tumor heterogeneity for studies on the biology and therapy of cancer metastasis. *Biochim. Biophys. Acta*, 651:37–50.
55. Hayward, W.S., Neel, B.G., and Astrin, S.M. (1981): Activation of a cellular *onc* gene by promoter insertion of ALV-induced lymphoid leukosis. *Nature*, 290:475–480.
56. Heisterkamp, N., Stephenson, J.R., Groffen, J., Hansen, P.F., deKlein, A., Bartram, C.R., and Grosveld, G. (1983): Localization of the c-*abl* oncogene adjacent to a translocation breakpoint in chronic myelocytic leukemia. *Nature*, 306:239–242.
57. Heppner, G.H. (1984): Tumor heterogeneity. *Cancer Res.*, 44:2259–2265.
58. Heppner, G.H., Loveless, S.E., Miller, M.F.R., Mahoney, K.H., and Fulton, A.M. (1984): Mammary tumor heterogeneity. In: *Cancer Invasion and Metastasis: Biologic and Therapeutic Aspects*, edited by G.L. Nicolson and L. Milas, pp. 209–221. Raven Press, New York.
59. Heppner, G.H., and Miller, B.E. (1983): Tumor heterogeneity: biological implications and therapeutic consequences. *Cancer Metastasis Rev.*, 2:5–23.
60. Herlyn, M., Balaban, G., Bennicelli, J., Guerry, D., Halaban, R., Herlyn, D., Elder, D.E., Maul, G.G., Steplewski, Z., Nowell, P.C., Clark, W.H., and Koprowski, H. (1985): Primary melanoma cells of the vertical growth phase: similarities to metastatic cells. *J. Natl. Cancer Inst.*, 74:283–289.
61. Hill, R.P., Chambers, A.F., Ling, V., and Harris, J.F. (1984): Dynamic heterogeneity: Rapid generation of metastatic variants in mouse B16 melanoma cells. *Science*, 224:998–1001.
62. Hunter, T. (1984): The proteins of oncogenes. *Sci. Am.*, 251:70–79.
63. Jones, P.D., and Taylor, S.M. (1980): Cellular differentiation, cytidine analogs, and DNA methylation. *Cell*, 2:85–93.
64. Katzav, S., Segal, S., and Feldman, M. (1985): Metastatic capacity of cloned T10 sarcoma cells that differ in H-2 expression: Inverse relationship to their immunogenic potency. *J. Natl. Cancer Inst.*, 75:307–318.
65. Kerbel, R.S., Frost, P., Liteplo, R., Carlow, D., and Elliott, B.E. (1984): Possible epigenetic mechanisms of tumor progression: Induction of high-frequency heritable but phenotypically unstable changes in the tumorigenic and metastatic properties of tumor cell populations by 5-azacytidine treatment. *J. Cell. Physiol.*, 3:87–97.
66. Klein, G. (1981): The role of gene dosage and genetic transpositions in carcinogenesis. *Nature*, 294:313–318.
67. Klein, G., ed. (1982): *Advances in Viral Oncology, Vol. x. The Transformation-Associated Cellular p53 Protein*. Raven Press, New York.
68. Klein, G. (1983): Specific chromosomal translocations and the genesis of B-cell-derived tumors in mice and men. *Cell*, 32:311–315.

69. Klein, G., and Klein, E. (1985): Evolution of tumours and the impact of molecular oncology. *Science*, 315:190–195.
70. Knudson, A.G., Jr. (1973): Mutation and human cancer. *Adv. Cancer Res.*, 17:317–352.
71. Knudson, A.G., Jr. (1985): Heredity cancer, oncogenes, and antioncogenes. *Cancer Res.*, 45:1437–1443.
72. Kris, R.M., Avivi, A., Bar-Eli, M., Alon, Y., Carmi, P., Schlessinger, J., and Raz, A. (1985): Expression of Ki-*ras* oncogene in tumor cell variants exhibiting different metastatic capabilities. *Int. J. Cancer*, 35:227–230.
73. Krontiris, T., and Cooper, G.M. (1981): Transforming activity of human tumor DNAs. *Proc. Natl. Acad. Sci. U.S.A.*, 78:1181–1184.
74. Kusyk, J.J., Seski, J.C., Medlin, V., and Edwards, C.L. (1981): Progressive chromosome changes associated with different sites of one ovarian carcinoma. *J. Natl. Cancer Inst.*, 66:1021–1025.
75. Lagarde, A.E., Donaghue, T.P., Dennis, J.W., and Kerbel, R.S. (1983): Genotypic and phenotypic evolution of a murine tumor during its progression in vivo toward metastasis. *J. Natl. Cancer Inst.*, 71:183–191.
76. Land, H., Parada, L.F., and Weinberg, R.A. (1983): Tumorigenic conversion of primary embryo fibroblasts requires at least two cooperating oncogenes. *Nature*, 304:596–601.
77. Landau, T., and Sachs, L. (1971): Characterization of the inducer required for the development of macrophage and granulocyte colonies. *Proc. Natl. Acad. Sci. U.S.A.*, 68:2540–2544.
78. Lane, M.A., Sainten, A., and Cooper, G.M. (1982): Stage specific transforming genes of human and mouse B- and T-lymphocyte neoplasms. *Cell*, 28:873–880.
79. Levin, G., and Mitelman, F. (1976): G-banding in Rous rat sarcomas during serial transfer: Significant chromosome observations and incidence of stromal mitoses. *Hereditas*, 84:1–14.
80. Ling, V., Chambers, A.F., Harris, J.F., and Hill, R.P. (1985): Quantitative genetic analysis of tumor progression. *Cancer Metastasis Rev.*, 4:173–194.
81. Little, C.D., Nau, M.M., Carney, D.N., Gazdar, A.F., and Minna, J.D. (1983): Amplification and expression of the c-*myc* oncogene in human lung cancer cell lines. *Nature*, 306:194–196.
82. Lotan, R., and Nicolson, G.L. (1979): Heterogeneity in growth inhibition by α-*trans*-retinoic acid of metastatic B16 melanoma clones and *in vivo*-selected cell variant lines. *Cancer Res.*, 39:4767–4771.
83. Metcalf, D. (1969): Studies on colony formation *in vitro* by mouse bone marrow cells. I. Continuous cluster formation and relation of clusters to colonies. *J. Cell. Physiol.*, 74:323–332.
84. Miller, B.E., Miller, F.R., and Heppner, G.H. (1981): Interactions between tumor subpopulations affecting their sensitivity to the antineoplastic agents cyclophosphamide and methotrexate. *Cancer Res.*, 41:4378–4381.
85. Miller, B.E., Miller, F.R., Leith, J., and Heppner, G.H. (1980): Growth interaction *in vivo* between tumor subpopulations derived from a single mouse mammary tumor. *Cancer Res.*, 40:3977–3981.
86. Miner, K.M., Kawaguchi, T., Uba, G.W., and Nicolson, G.L. (1982): Clonal drift of cell surface, melanogenic and experimental properties of *in vivo*-selected, brain meninges-colonizing murine B16 melanoma. *Cancer Res.*, 42:4631–4638.
87. Mintz, B., and Illmensee, K. (1975): Normal genetically mosaic mice produced from malignant teratocarcinoma cells. *Proc. Natl. Acad. Sci. U.S.A.*, 72:3585–3589.
88. Muller, R., Slamon, D.J., Tremblay, J.M., Cline, M.J., and Verma, I.M. (1982): Differential expression of cellular oncogenes during pre- and postnatal development of the mouse. *Nature*, 299:640–643.
89. Murray, M.J., Cunningham, J.M., Parada, L.F., Dautry, F., Lebowitz, P., and Weinberg, R.A. (1983): The HL-60 transforming sequence: A *ras* oncogene coexisting with altered *myc* genes in hematopoietic tumors. *Cell*, 33:749–757.
90. Nepreu, A., Fahrlander, P.O., Yang, J.Q., and Marcu, K.B. (1985): Amplification and altered expression of the c-*myc* oncogene in A-MuLV-transformed fibroblasts. *Nature*, 317:440–443.
91. Newbold, R.F., and Overall, R.W. (1983): Fibroblast, immortality is a prerequisite for transformation by EJ c-Ha-*ras* oncogene. *Nature*, 304:648–651.
92. Nicolson, G.L. (1982): Cancer metastasis: Organ colonization and the cell surface properties of malignant cells. *Biochim. Biophys. Acta*, 695:113–176.
93. Nicolson, G.L. (1984): Cell surface molecules and tumor metastasis. Regulation of metastatic diversity. *Exp. Cell Res.*, 150:3–22.
94. Nicolson, G.L. (1984): Generation of phenotypic diversity and progression in metastatic tumors. *Cancer Metastasis Rev.*, 3:25–42.

95. Nicolson, G.L. (1984): Tumor progression, oncogenes and the evolution of metastatic phenotypic diversity. *Clin. Exp. Metastasis,* 2:85–105.
96. Nicolson, G.L., and Poste, G. (1982): Tumor cell diversity and host responses in cancer metastasis. I. Properties of metastatic cells. *Curr. Probl. Cancer* 7(6):1–83.
97. Nicolson, G.L., and Poste, G. (1983): Tumor cell diversity and host responses in cancer metastasis. II. Host immune responses and therapy of metastases. *Curr. Probl. Cancer,* 7(7):1–43.
98. Nicolson, G.L., and Poste, G. (1983): Tumor implantation and invasion at metastatic sites. *Int. Rev. Exp. Pathol.,* 25:77–181.
99. Nicolson, G.L., Rotter, V., Wolf, D., Irimura, T., Reading, C.L., La Biche, R., and Frazier, M. (1986): Biochemistry and molecular biology of RAW117 large-cell lymphoma. In: *Biochemistry and Molecular Genetics of Cancer Metastasis,* edited by F.K. Lapis, L.A. Liotta, and A.S. Rabson, pp. 115–127. Martinus Nijhoff/Dr. W. Junk Publisher, Hingham, Massachusetts.
100. Nowell, P.C. (1976): The clonal evolution of tumor cell populations. *Science,* 194:23–28.
101. Nowell, P.C. (1983): Tumor progression and clonal evolution: The role of genetic instability. In: *Chromosome Mutation and Neoplasia,* edited by J. German, pp. 413–432. Alan R. Liss, Inc., New York.
102. Nowell, P.C., and Balaban, G. (1985): Karyotypic progression and metastasis formation of human tumors. In: *Biochemistry and Molecular Genetics of Cancer Metastasis,* edited by F.K. Lapis, L.A. Liotta, and A.S. Rabson, pp. 129–136. Martinus Nijhoff/Dr. W. Junk Publishers, Hingham, Massachusetts.
103. Nusse, R., and Varmus, H.E. (1982): Many tumors induced by the mouse mammary tumor virus contain a provirus integrated in the same region of the host genome. *Cell,* 31:99–109.
104. Ozanne, B., Wheeler, T., Zack, J., Smith, G., and Dale, B. (1982): Transforming gene of a human leukaemia cell is unrelated to the expressed tumor virus-related gene of the cell. *Nature,* 299:744–747.
105. Paget, S. (1889): The distribution of secondary growth in cancer of the breast. *Lancet,* 1:571–573.
106. Payne, G.S., Bishop, J.M., and Varmus, H.E. (1982): Multiple arrangements of viral DNA and an activated host oncogene in bursal lymphomas. *Nature,* 295:209–214.
107. Pearce, V., Pathak, S., Mellard, D., Welch, D.R., and Nicolson, G.L. (1984): Chromosome and DNA analysis of rat 13762NF mammary adenocarcinoma cell lines and clones of different metastatic potentials. *Clin. Exp. Metastasis,* 2:271–286.
108. Peters, G., Brookes, S., Smith, R., and Dickson, C. (1983): Tumorigenesis by mouse mammary tumor virus: Evidence for a common region for provirus integration in mammary tumors. *Cell,* 33:369–377.
109. Peterson, J.A., Bartholomew, J.C., Stampfer, M., and Ceriani, R.L. (1981): Analysis of expression of human mammary epithelial antigens in normal and malignant breast cells at the single cell level by flow cytofluorimetry. *Exp. Cell Biol.,* 49:1–14.
110. Peterson, J.A., Ceriani, R.L., Blank, E.W., Osvaldo, L. (1983): Comparison of rates of phenotypic variability in surface antigen expression in normal and cancerous breast epithelial cells. *Cancer Res.,* 43:4291–4296.
111. Pierce, G.B., Lewis, S.H., Miller, G.J., Motitz, E., and Miller, P. (1979): Tumorigenicity of embryonal carcinoma as an assay to study control of malignancy blastocyst. *Proc. Natl. Acad. Sci. U.S.A.,* 76:6649–6655.
112. Poste, G. (1982): Experimental systems for analysis of the malignant phenotype. *Cancer Metastasis Rev.,* 1:141–199.
113. Poste, G., Doll, J., and Fidler, I.J. (1981): Interactions among local subpoulations affects stability of the metastatic phenotype in polyclonal populations of B16 melanoma cells. *Proc. Natl. Acad. Sci. U.S.A.,* 78:6226–6230.
114. Poste, G., and Greig, R. (1982): On the genesis and regulation of cellular heterogeneity in malignant tumors. *Invasion and Metastasis,* 2:137–176.
115. Poste, G., Greig, R., Tzeng, J., Koestler, T., and Corwin, S. (1984): Interactions between tumor-cell subpopulations in malignant tumors. In: *Cancer Invasion and Metastasis: Biologic and Therapeutic,* edited by G.L. Nicolson and L. Milas. pp. 223–243. Raven Press, New York.
116. Pulciani, S., Santos, E., Lauver, A.V., Long, L.K., and Barbacid, M. (1982): Oncogenes in solid human tumors. *Nature,* 300:539–542.
117. Razin, A., and Riggs, A. (1980): DNA methylation and gene function. *Science,* 210:604–610.
118. Reading, C.L., Brunson, K.W., Torriani, M., and Nicolson, G.L. (1980): Malignancies of metastatic murine lymphosarcoma cell lines and clones correlate with decreased cell surface display of RNA tumor virus envelope glycoprotein gp70. *Proc. Natl. Acad. Sci. U.S.A.,* 77:5943–5947.

119. Reddy, E.P., Reynolds, R.K., Santos, E., and Barbacid, M. (1982): A point mutation is responsible for the acquisition of transforming properties of the T24 human bladder carcinoma oncogene. *Nature*, 300:149–152.

120. Rotter, V., Wolf, D., Blick, M., and Nicolson, G.L. (1985): Expression of *abl* and other oncogenes is independent of metastatic potential in Abelson virus-transformed malignant murine large-cell lymphoma. *Clin. Exp. Metastasis*, 3:77–86.

121. Rotter, V., Wolf, D., and Nicolson, G.L. (1984): The expression of transformation-related protein p53- and p53-containing mRNA in murine RAW117 large-cell lymphoma cells of differing metastatic potential. *Clin. Exp. Metastasis*, 2:199–204.

122. Rowley, J.D. (1983): Human oncogene locations and chromosome aberrations. *Nature*, 301:290–291.

123. Rubin, H. (1985): Cancer as a dynamic developmental disorder. *Cancer Res.*, 45:2935–2942.

124. Ruley, H.E. (1983): Adenovirus early region IA enables viral and cellular transforming genes to transform primary cells in culture. *Nature*, 304:602–606.

125. Sachs, L. (1980): Constitutive uncoupling of pathways of gene expression that control growth and differentiation in myeloid: A model for the origin and progression of malignancy. *Proc. Natl. Acad. Sci. U.S.A.*, 77:6152–6156.

126. Sager, R., Tanaka, K., Lau, C.C., Ebina, W., and Anisowicz, A. (1983): Resistance of human cell to tumorigenesis induced by cloned transforming genes. *Proc. Natl. Acad. Sci. U.S.A.*, 80:7601–7605.

127. Schirrmacher, V. (1985): Cancer metastasis: Experimental approaches, theoretical concepts, and treatment strategies. *Adv. Cancer Res.*, 43:1–73.

128. Schwab, M., Varmus, H.E., Bishop, J.M., Grzeschik, K.H., Naylor, S.L., Sakaguchi, A.Y., Brodeur, G., and Trent, J. (1984): Chromosome localization in normal human cells and neuroblastoma of a gene related to c-*myc*. *Nature*, 308:288–91.

129. Shih, C., Shilo, B.-Z., Goldfarb, M.P., Dannenberg, A., Weinberg, R. (1979): Passage of phenotypes of chemically transformed cells via transfection of DNA and chromatin. *Proc. Natl. Acad. Sci. U.S.A.*, 76:5714–5718.

130. Shiosaka, T., and Saunders, G.F. (1982): Differential expression of selected genes in human leukemia leukocytes. *Proc. Natl. Acad. Sci. U.S.A.*, 79:4668–4671.

131. Slamon, D.J., DeKernion, J.B., Verma, I.M., and Cline, M.J. (1984): Expression of cellular oncogenes in human malignancies. *Science*, 224:256–262.

132. Stackpole, C.W. (1983): Generation of phenotypic diversity in the B16 mouse melanoma relative to spontaneous metastasis. *Cancer Res.*, 43:3057–3065.

133. Stanbridge, E.J. (1985): A case for human tumor-suppressor genes. *Bioessays (in press)*.

134. Sukumar, S., Notario, V., Martin-Zanca, D., and Barbacid, M. (1983): Induction of mammary carcinomas in rats by nitrosomethylurea involves malignant activation of H-*ras*-1 locus by single point mutations. *Nature*, 306:658–661.

135. Sukumar, S., Pulciani, S., Doniger, J., DiPaolo, J.A., Evans, C.H., Zbar, B., and Barbacid, M. (1984): A transforming *ras* gene in tumorigenic guinea pig cell lines initiated by diverse chemical carcinogens. *Science*, 223:1197–1199.

136. Tabin, C.J., Bradley, S.M., Bargmann, C.I., Weinberg, R.A., Papageorge, A.G., Scolnick, E.M., Dhar, R., Chang, L., and Chang, E.H. (1982): Mechanism of activation of a human oncogene. *Nature*, 300:143–149.

137. Tainsky, M.A., Cooper, C.S., Giovanella, B.C., and Vande Woude, G.F. (1984): An activated *ras*^N gene: Detected in late but not early passage human PA1 teratocarcinoma cells. *Science*, 225:643–645.

138. Talmadge, J.E., Talmadge, C.B., Zbar, B., McEwen, R., and Meeker, A.K. (1986): *submitted*.

139. Taub, R., Moulding, C., Battey, J., Murphy, W., Vasicek, T., Lenoir, G.M., and Leder, P. (1984): Activation and somatic mutation of the translocated c-*myc* gene in Burkitt lymphoma cells. *Cell*, 36:399–348.

140. Temin, H.M. (1984): Do we understand the genetic mechanism of oncogenesis? *J. Cell. Physiol. [Suppl.]*, 3:1–11.

141. Testa, J.R., Mintz, U., Rowly, J.E., Vardiman, J.W., and Golomb, H.M. (1979): Evolution of karyotypes in active nonlymphatic leukemia. *Cancer Res.*, 39:3619–3627.

142. Thor, A., Horan Hand, P., Wunderlich, D., Caruso, A., and Muraro, R. (1984): Monoclonal antibodies define differential *ras* gene expression in malignant and benign colonic diseases. *Nature*, 311:562–565.

143. Thorgeirsson, U.P., Turpeenniemi-Hujanen, T., Williams, J.E., Westin, E.H., Heilman, C.A., Talmadge, J.E., and Liotta, L.A. (1985): NIH/3T3 cells transfected with human tumor DNA

containing activated *ras* on oncogenes express the metastatic phenotype in nude mice. *Mole. Cell Biol.,* 5:259–262.

144. Thorgeirsson, U.P., Turpeenniemi-Hujanen, T., Talmadge, J.E., and Liotta, L.A. (1986): Expression of oncogenes in cancer metastase In: *Cancer Metastasis: Experimental and Clinical Strategies,* edited by D.R. Welch, B.K. Bhuyan, and L.A. Liotta, pp. 77–93. Alan R. Liss, New York.

145. Tsuruo, T., and Fidler, I.J. (1981): Differences in drug sensitivity among tumor cells from parental tumors, selected variants, and spontaneous metastases. *Cancer Res.,* 41:3058–3064.

146. Varmus, H. (1984): The molecular genetics of cellular oncogenes. *Annu. Rev. Genet.,* 18:553–612.

147. Vousden, K.H., and Marshall, D.J. (1984): Three different activated *ras* genes in mouse tumors: Evidence for oncogene activation during progression of a mouse lymphoma. *EMBO J.,* 3:913–917.

148. Weinberg, R.A. (1982): Oncogenes of spontaneous and chemically induced tumors. *Adv. Cancer Res.,* 36:149–164.

149. Weinberg, R.A. (1983): A molecular basis of cancer. *Sci. Am.,* 249:126–143.

150. Weiner, F., Ohno, S., Babonits, M., Sumegi, J., Wirschursky, Z., Klein, G., Mushinski, J.F., and Potter, M. (1984): Hemizygous interstitial deletion of chromosome 15 (band D) in three plasmacytomas). *Proc. Natl. Acad. Sci. U.S.A.,* 81:1159–1163.

151. Weiss, L. (1983): Random and nonrandom processes in metastasis, and metastatic efficiency. *Invasion and Metastasis,* 3:193–208.

152. Welch, D.R., Evans, D.P., Tomasovic, S.P., Milas, L., and Nicolson, G.L. (1984): Multiple phenotypic divergence of mammary adenocarcinoma cell clones. II. Sensitivity to radiation, hyperthemia and FUdR. *Clin. Exp. Metastasis,* 2:357–371.

153. Welch, D.R., Krizman, D., and Nicolson, G.L. (1984): Multiple phenotypic divergence of mammary adenocarcinoma cell clones. I. *In vitro* and *in vivo* properties. *Clin. Exp. Metastasis,* 2:333–355.

154. Westin, E.H., Wong-Staal, F., Gelmann, E.P., Favera, R.D., Papas, T.S., Lautenberger, J.A., Eva, A., Reddy, E.P., Tronick, S.R., Aaronson, S.A., and Gallo, R.C. (1982): Expression of cellular homologous of retroviral *onc* genes in human hematopoietic cells. *Proc. Natl. Acad. Sci. U.S.A.,* 79:2490–2494.

155. Wolman, S.R. (1983): Karyotypic progression in human tumors. *Cancer Metastasis Rev.,* 2:257–293.

156. Yuasa, Y., Gol, R.A., Chang, A., Chin, I.-M., Reddy, E.P., Tronick, S.R., and Aaronson, S.A. (1984): Mechanism of activation of an N-*ras* oncogene of SW-1271 human lung carcinoma cells. *Proc. Natl. Acad. Sci. U.S.A.,* 81:3670–3674.

157. Yuasa, Y., Srivastava, S.K., Dunn, C.Y., Rhim, J.S., Reddy, E.P., Aaronson, S.A. (1983): Acquisition of transforming properties by alternative point mutations within c-*bas/has* human neoplasia. *Nature,* 303:775–779.

Subject Index

A

2-T antigen virus, 26–28
75-kD tumor-associated antigen
  human nerve growth factor receptor,
    86–87
  properties, 86
abl-coded p160
  phosphorylation, 148–149
  synthesis, 148–149
Actin, 59–60
AEV, v-*erb*-B, 55
AEV-R
  erb-A, 53–54
  erb-B, 53–54
  genetic structure, 53
  protein products, 63–64
Allele
  autonomously oncogenic mutant, 64
  inhibitor, Rb-1, 104–105
  normal, 45
  transduced mutant, 45
Amino acid sequence
  c-*mos*^{ch}, 76–77
  c-*mos*^{hu}, 76–77
  c-*mos*^{mu}, 76–77
Antigen loss, 154
Avian acute leukemia virus, 46
Avian carcinoma virus MH2, 46
Avian erythroblastosis virus strain R, 46

B

Baby rat kidney cell, 2
Basal epithelial cell, 32
Bovine papillomavirus type 1, 30–32
  genetic map, 27
BPV1 DNA, 37
BPV1 DNA transfection, stepwise trans-
  formation, 34–38

C

C-11 revertant, 117–122
  biological properties, 119
  culture fluid, 119
  functional classification, 121
  molecular properties, 119
  target-deficient, 121
  target-related, 119–120
  v-Ki-*ras* genome, 118–119
Ca antigen, 86–87
Cancer
  naturally occurring, 97
  papillomavirus, 32–33
Cell fusion, 120
  experiment, 115
Cell hybrid, human intraspecies, tumor
    suppression, 89
Cell morphology, 143–144
Cell surface antigen, 143–144
Cell transformation, DNA virus, 21
Cellular gene, oncogene inhibition,
  103–122
c-*erb*-A, 55–56
c-Ha-*ras* mRNA level, 94
c-Ha-*ras* p21 protein level, 95
c-Ha-*ras* proto-oncogene, 108
Chicken c-*myc,* 47–49
Chromosome
  breakage, 140
  instability, 83
  number increase, 157
  rearrangement, 146
  segregation, malignancy reversion,
    137–138
  stability, 83
    human hybrid cell, 83
CMII, 49–51
c-*mos*
  chicken, 71–79
  human, 71–79
  mouse, 71–79
c-*mos*^{ch}
  activation, 77
  amino acid sequence comparison, 77
c-*mos*^{hu}
  activation, 73–74
  biological activity, 74
  regulatory sequence, 73–74
  structure, 74

c-*mos*^mu, expression, 78
c-*myc* gene, 2
c-*myc*^N, amplification, 151
Colony-stimulating factor, 129–130
c-*onc* gene, 45, 146, 149
    amplification, 150–151
    heterogenous expression, 149–150
Cotransduced sequence, single hybrid
        protein, 56–63
Cotransduction, 53
    proto-oncogene, 64
Cotransfection, 2
    ElA, 2
c-*ras*, 147
CSF-1 receptor, 41

D

Dermis fibroblast, 32
Differentiation, different pathway,
        135–137
Differentiation clone, 133–135
Differentiation factor, 129–132
    induction, 133–135
    uncoupling, 132–133
Diploid human fibroblast, suppression
        transformation, 105
DMN 4A, 105
DNA methylation, 159–160
DNA sequence, 106
DNA transfection/transformation assay,
        148
DNA tumor virus
    cooperative interactions, 21–37
    stepwise transformation, 21–37
DNA virus, cell transformation, 21

E
ElA, 2
    DNA replication, 7–9
    mutant, 6–7
    mutant gene, 5–6
    plasmid, 5–9
    protein coding sequence, 5
    T24 Ha-*ras*, 5, 7
    transcription, 6, 7–9
    transforming functions, 5–9
    translation products, 6
ElA protein, biological activity, 7
ElB, 2
E26
    ets, 57–59

genetic structure, 57
hybrid protein, 64
myb, 57–59
Early protein, 32
env, 45
erb-A, 53–54
erb-B, 53–54
Erythroleukemic cell, 135
Erythroprotein, 135
ES4, 46
ets, 57–59

F
F-2, target deficient, 121
F-2 revertant, 117–122
    biological properties, 119
    culture fluid, 119
    functional classification, 121
    molecular properties, 119
    target-related, 119–120
    v-Ki-*ras* genome, 118–119
FBR-MSV
    fos, 60–61
    fox, 60–61
    genetic structure, 60–61
    hybrid protein, 64
fes
    C-11 revertant, 120–121
    F-2 revertant, 120–121
fgr, 59–60
fms oncogene, 71
fox, 60–61
FR3T3 derivative, BPV1-transformed,
        34–36

G
G418-resistant colony, 11, 13
gag, 45, 47
Gene dosage, 115, 138
Gene expression
    biochemical analysis, 63–64
    genetic analysis, 63–64
    metastatic cell, 153–154
Genetic cooperation, 29–30
Genetic defect, bypassing, 137–138
Genetic instability, 143–162
Genetic regulation, somatic cell hybrid,
        83–98
Genome
    polyomavirus, 22–28
    retroviral, 45–64

Genome *(cont.)*
    structure
        biochemical analysis, 63–64
        genetic analysis, 63–64
    vertical transmission, 21
Genomic instability, tumor progression,
    154–157
Granulocyte inducer, 129–130
GR-FeSV
    actin, 59–60
    fgr, 59–60
    genetic structure, 59
    hybrid protein, 64
Growth factor, 109, 117
    normal, 129–132
    receptor, 109, 117
    uncoupling, 132–133

H
HaPV, 22
Ha-*ras* oncogene, 2
Hematopoietic cell, growth and differenti-
    ation factors, 130–132
HPV DNA, 32–33
HPVla, genetic map, 27
HPV6 DNA, 32
HPV11 DNA, 33
HPV16 DNA, 33
hrl, 5–6, 8–9
HT1080 human fibrosarcoma cell, 89
    N-*ras* gene, 91–92
Human adenovirus, 1
Human bladder carcinoma cell line EJ,
    93–94
Human chorionic gonadotrophin, alpha
    subunit, 87
Human diploid fibroblast, 89, 115
Human fibroblast, 88
Human papillomavirus, 30–32
Hybrid cell
    oncogene expression, 91–94
    segregant. See Segregant hybrid cell
    somatic. See Somatic hybrid cell
    tumor suppression, 91–94
Hybrid c-*mos*^mu/c-*mos*^hu gene, 74–75

I
Immortality, 23
Immortalization gene, 115

K
Keratinocyte, 32

L
Large T protein, 24–25
    intracellular localization, 28
Long terminal repeat, 71
LTR-activated c-*mos*
    biological transforming activity, 71
    transcription regulatory element, 71
LTR enhancer sequence, 71

M
Macrophage inducer, 129–130
Malignancy
    development, 129–139
    suppression, 129–139
        specific chromosome association,
            87–91
MC29, 49–51
    v-*myc* oncogene, 2
Metaphase chromosome, 96
Metastatic phenotype, evolution, 143–162
Metastasis
    gene expression, 153–154
    oncogene, 151–153
MH2, 46
    gag, 47, 49
    genetic structure, 47
    mil, 47–53
    myc, 47–53
    protein products, 63–64
    v-*mil*, 49, 51
    v-*myc*, 49–52
MH2E21, genetic structure, 50–51
MH2E21ml, genetic structure, 50–51
Microcell transfer, 96
Microenvironment, 144–145, 160–161
Middle I protein, 23–26
mil, 47–53
mos oncogene, 71–79
mos proto-oncogene, 71, 78
mos transforming efficiency, 74–75
myb, 57–59
myc, 47–53
Myeloid cell, 129–132
Myeloid leukemic cell, 133
    clone classification, 134
    mutant, 137
Myeloid precursor cell, 130–132
    differentiation, 136

N
Neoplastic state, subthreshold, 36
Neoplastic transformation, oncogene,
    145–148
Neuroblastoma, 104
NIH/3T3
    biological properties, 119
    doubly transformed, 117–118
        biological properties, 118
        ouabain, 117–118
        ras oncogene, 118
    molecular properties, 119
NIH/3T3 cell, 72–73, 91–92
    Ki-*ras*-transformed, 117–122

O
OK10, 49–51
Oncogene
    active, 45
    biochemical functions, 17
    cell transformation, 1
        complementing oncogene, 1–17
    cellular, transduced mutant allele, 45
    cloned, 1
    complementation, 1–5
    defined, 1
    expression, hybrid cell, 91–94
    gene structure, 1
    immunological study, 109
    inhibition, cellular gene, 103–122
    interactions, 17
    mechanism, 1
    metabolic pathway, 1
    metastasis, 151–153
    molecular analysis, 108–109
    neoplastic transformation, 145–148
    product, molecular analysis, 108–109
    stage-specific, 29–30
    transformation, 17
    tumor progression, 148--154
Oncogene complementation analysis,
    1–17
Ouabain, 117–118, 122

P
p21, 150
p53 tumor antigen, cell transformation, 28
Papilloma, 32
    host range, 32
Papillomavirus, 21
    cancer, 32–33

genetic organization, 27
stepwise transformation, 30–36
tumor progression, 30–36
Phenotype
    diversification
        epigenetic effects, 159–160
        rate, 158
    instability, 157–161
    malignant, oncogene complementation
        analysis, 1–17
    metastatic evolution, 143–162
    revertant, origin, 111–115
    transformed
        naturally occurring resistance,
            104–105
        pathway, 107
        tumorigenic, 84–87
Pleiotropic gene complex, 21
pmt, 5
pol, 45
Polyoma, 22–26
    genetic map, 27
Polyoma virus, 1, 21
    genome, 22–28
    multiple oncogene, 22–28
    paradigms, 29–30
Polyoma virus early region, 2
Polyoma virus large T antigen, 2
Polyoma virus middle T antigen, 2
Polyoma virus protein, 22–23
Propagation, horizontal, 21
Protein
    early, 32
    single hybrid, 56–63
Proto-oncogene, 45
    analysis, 107–108
    cotransduction, 64
    expression, 107–108, 145
    lower organism, 108
    retroviral oncogene, 107–108
    structure, 145
Proviral transcription element, 71
Provirus, 106

R
R5-5-1 revertant, 116–117
ras, C-11 revertant, 120–121
ras gene, 2
    myb, 5
    N-*myc*, 5
    p53, 5

ras oncogene, 2, 109
  REF52 cell, 15
ras p21
  REF52 cell, 15
Rat embryo fibroblast cell, 2
Rat fibroblast cell, properties, 24
REF cell, 36–37
REF52
  ras p21, 15
  stepwise transformation, 10, 12
  T24 Ha-*ras* expression, 10, 14
  transformed clone outgrowth, 10, 13
REF52 cell
  E1A, 9
  morphology, 10, 14
  multistep transformation, 9–14
  ras gene, 9
  ras oncogene, 15
Re-revertant cell, 137–138
Resistant cell, isolation, 109–111
Restriction-fragment-length polymor-
    phism, 89–90
Retinoblastoma
  hereditary, 104
  nonhereditary, 104
Retransformation, resist, 120
Retroviral genome, single, multiple-cell-
    derived sequences, 45–64
Retroviral oncogene, 45
  function, 107–109
  molecular analysis, 106–107
  pathway, 107
  product, function, 107–109
  proto-oncogene, 107–108
  transformation cell resistance, 109–122
Retroviral v-*myc* allele, 47–49
Revertant cell
  C-11, 117–122
    biological properties, 119
    culture fluid, 119
    functional classification, 121
    molecular properties, 119
    target deficient, 121
    target-related, 119–120
    v-Ki-*ras* genome, 118–119
  classification, 113–115
  early studies, 116
  F-2
    biological properties, 119
    culture fluid, 119
    functional classification, 121
    molecular properties, 119
    target deficient, 121

    target related, 119–120
    v-Ki-*ras* genome, 118–119
  frequency of occurrence, 109–122
  oncogene-altered, 113–114
  oncoprotein-deficient, 113–114
  ouabain, 110–111
  properties, 116–122
  R5-5-1, 116–117
  target-deficient, 113–115, 121
  target-related, 113–114, 117–122
Rodent embryo fibroblast, 23
RSV
  genetic structure, 61–62
  hybrid protein, 64
  src, 61–63
  src', 61–63

S
Sarcoma, 137–138
  chromosome segregation, 138
Segregant hybrid cell
  historical aspects, 83–84
  phenotypic characteristics, 85
  transformed, 84–87
  tumorigenic, 88–89
    phenotype, 84–87
Sequence, multiple-cell-derived, 45–64
Somatic cell hybrid
  chromosomal instability, 83
  tumor genetic regulation, 83–98
Soncogene, 137–138
src', 61–63
  C-11 revertant, 120–121
  F-2 revertant, 120–121
Stepwise transformation, 29
  BPV1 DNA transfection, 34–38
  papillomavirus, 30–36
Suppression transformation, diploid
    human fibroblast, 105
SV40, 26–28
  genetic map, 27
  transformed, biological properties, 26

T
T24, Ha-*ras,* 5–6, 8–9
  E1A, 5, 7
Target gene, 112–113
  altered, 113
  target deficient, 113
Transcription regulator, 72–73
Transcription terminator, 71

Transfection assay, 147–148
Transfection technique, DNA-mediated, 122
Transformation
  biochemical pathway, 103
  genetic resistance, 103–122
  oncogene, 17
  p53 tumor antigen, 28
  quantitative aspects, 115
Transformation resistant cell, 109–122
  frequency of occurrence, 110
  ouabain, 110–111
Transmission, vertical, 21
Tropomyosin, 121–122
Tumor cell, microenvironment, 144–145
Tumor cell heterogeneity, 143–145
  origin, 144
Tumor progression, 23, 26
  chromosome change, 156
  genetic instability, 154–157
  microenvironment, 160–161
  oncogene, 148–158
  papillomavirus, 30–36
  phenotypic instability, 157–161
  rate, 144

Tumor suppression, 129–139
  biological nature, 91
  hybrid cell, 91–94
Tumor-suppressor gene
  molecular identification, 95–97
  naturally occurring cancer, 97
  oncogene, 97

U
Upstream mouse sequence, 71–73
  c-*mos*^{mu}, 72–73
  v-*mos*, 72–73

V
v-*erb*-B, 55
v-*erb*-B allele, 55–56
Virus, 3-T antigen, 22–26
v-Ki-*ras*, 120
v-*mil*, v-*raf*, 51
v-*onc* gene, 45

W
Wilms' tumor, 104